HEIDELBERG SCIENCE LIBRARY | Volume 8

The Pharmacology of Psychotherapeutic Drugs

F. Th. v. Brücke · O. Hornykiewicz · E. B. Sigg

Springer-Verlag Berlin Heidelberg GmbH | 1969

First published in 1966

F. Th. v. Brücke und O. Hornykiewicz
„Pharmakologie der Psychopharmaka"

Translated and revised by Ernest B. Sigg

© by Springer-Verlag Berlin Heidelberg 1969
Softcover reprint of the hardcover 1st edition 1969
Library of Congress Catalog Card Number 72-90045

ISBN 978-0-387-90009-4   ISBN 978-1-4615-8047-8 (eBook)
DOI 10.1007/978-1-4615-8047-8

Title No. 3917

Contents

Introduction

According to Roth (1964), the term "psychopharmakon" was used for the first time by Reinhardus Lorichius of Hadamar who, in 1548, edited a collection of prayers of comfort and in preparation for death under the title "Psychopharmakon, hoc est: medicina animae". With the introduction of chlorpromazine in 1952, the era of psychopharmacology began. The "psychopharmakon" of the Renaissance and the twentieth century differ from each other in concept and meaning; the spiritual support in times of increased anxiety and fear has been replaced by drugs which "tranquilize" the agitated and brighten the mood of the depressed. Thus, the pioneering discovery by Delay et al. (1952) of the usefulness of phenothiazines in schizophrenics, followed by the report of Loomer et al. (1957) on the antidepressant effect of iproniazid and Kuhn's (1957) observation of the thymoleptic property of imipramine triggered a revolution in psychiatry. Subsequently, numerous new psychopharmaka have been introduced. Parallel with this development, the interest in experimental behavioral research which began to utilize the newly discovered drugs as tools grew rapidly. The experience gained from studies of human and animal behavior found expression in the attempt to introduce a nomenclature and classify psychopharmaka on a purely psychological basis. Pharmacology followed this development only slowly. Nevertheless, it must be emphasized that all psychopharmaka have a distinct effect on the central and/or peripheral nervous system. Therefore, real progress in the understanding of the mechanism of action is only to be achieved if the effect of these agents on the physiology of these well defined substrates is studied, utilizing biochemical, psychological and electrophysiological methods.

The purpose of the present essay is to show the student that, in spite of the enormous difficulties encountered in CNS-research, significant advances have been made towards the understanding of the mechanism of action of psychopharmaka. This becomes particularly apparent if the various groups of centrally active agents are compared,

1

as has been successfully done in the review by E. Jacobsen in 1959. In this contribution we have emphasized the therapeutically useful classes of psychopharmaka, omitting a presentation of the oldest groups of "poisons" with psychotropic effects, the hallucinogens. For detailed information regarding methodology used to detect psychopharmacologically active agents, the reader is referred to the review of Riley and Spinks (1958).

In principle we have followed the recommendations of WHO in respect to nomenclature, and the "non-proprietary" (generic) names have been introduced according to the compilation of "Psychotropic Drugs and Related Compounds" by Usdin and Efron (1967). Their compendium as well as that edited by Pöldinger and Schmidlin (1963) also contain a complete listing of synonyms, trade names and structural formulae.

It is hoped that the present volume, though incomplete and restricted in scope, will be helpful for those who seek to understand the pharmacodynamics of psychotherapeutic drugs.

I. Phenothiazine Derivatives

Methylene blue, synthesized by Caro in 1876, is the first phenothiazine derivative for which effects on the CNS were described. It
possesses a mild hypnotic effect and prolongs the action of barbiturates (Konzett, 1938).

The introduction of chlorpromazine (CPZ) in 1950 was of great
importance. Laborit and Huguenard (1951, 1952) attempted to
influence cases of catatonia by inducing hypothermia with mixtures
of pharmaceutical preparations which among other constitutents
contained CPZ. However, the results of these experiments were
inconclusive Delay, Deniker and Harl (1952) noticed that in agitated
psychotic patients CPZ not only exerts a calming effect, but also
causes a change in affective behavior and drive. These authors
recognized for the first time the unique possibility for a symptomatic
pharmacotherapy of mental disorders.

Since the introduction of CPZ into the clinic, innumerable phenothiazine derivatives with similar pharmacologic and clinical profiles
of activities have become available to the clinician. A quantitative
comparison of the pharmacologic actions of a number of compounds
with CPZ-like effects is illustrated in the tables of this text.

A. Structure-activity Relationships

Variations of the most frequently used phenothiazines concern
substitutions at the 2-position of the phenothiazine nucleus, e. g.
halogen, methoxy, trifluormethane, acyl, methylmercapto or various
substituted sulfonamide groups, to mention the most important
possibilities.

Also important is the N-substituted side chain. If it is a N-dialkyl-
aminoalkyl side chain, it most often contains two or three carbon atoms.
The compounds with two carbon atom chains are frequently antihistaminics (promethazine) or cholinolytics (diethazine), whereas the
three carbon chain is typically found in neuroleptics (promazine).

3

Another group of phenothiazine derivatives contains a terminal piperidine ring (mepazine) which diminishes the central sedative component. A piperazine ring in the N-substituted side chain generally enhances extrapyramidal side-effects. However, the neuroleptic activity is also increased as evidenced by the smaller dose necessary to achieve therapeutic efficacy.

A complete survey of the phenothiazine literature, with particular consideration of the chemistry, was recently published by Schenker and Herbst (1963). (The publication contains one hundred and two tables with chemical structures and 6800 literature references.)

B. Peripheral Effects

Phenothiazines exert a variety of effects on peripheral organs and tissues. They influence the functions of the peripheral autonomic system, the vascular system and the striated musculature, as described in the now classical publication of Courvoisier et al. (1953). This was soon followed by reports of Huidobro (1954), Kopera and Armitage (1954), Ryall (1956), and Delga and Hazard (1957) on the peripheral effects of CPZ *in vivo* and *in vitro*. In many instances, the findings of Courvoisier et al. (1953) were confirmed and extended although some of their original data had to be corrected.

1. Adrenolytic, Cholinolytic, Antihistaminic and Anti-serotonin Effects

CPZ antagonizes the peripheral effects of epinephrine, acetylcholine, histamine and 5-hydroxytryptamine (5-HT, serotonin) *in vitro* and *in vivo*.

The adrenolytic effect of CPZ is particularly marked. Courvoisier et al. (1953) have found that practically all effects of epinephrine are blocked by CPZ. In the chloralose anesthetized dog the epinephrine effect on blood pressure is reversed after i. v. injection of 5 mg/kg of CPZ. The vasopressor effect of norepinephrine is diminished but never completely blocked or reversed. Moreover, the rise in blood pressure induced by bilateral carotid artery occlusion and by electrical stimulation of the central end of the cut vagus nerve is blocked by CPZ. Pretreatment of mice and rabbits with CPZ considerably diminishes the acute toxicity of epinephrine and norepinephrine. In this respect, CPZ is more potent than promethazine and dibenamine.

4

Epinephrine-evoked contractions of the isolated rabbit uterus (Courvoisier et al., 1953; Kopera and Armitage, 1954) or isolated aortic strips (Martin et al., 1960) are also blocked by CPZ. On the other hand, Courvoisier et al. (1953) did not observe any effect of CPZ on epinephrine-induced hyperglycemia in the rabbit. As a matter of fact, in this species CPZ *per se* causes a slight hyperglycemia. Martin et al. (1960) demonstrated that not all effects of epinephrine are diminished by CPZ. Thus, the vasopressor and positive chronotropic effects of norepinephrine (and, to some extent, epinephrine) are potentiated and prolonged by CPZ in the vagotomized, spinal cat. Martin et al. (1960) suggested that this effect is due to blockade by CPZ of an important mechanism responsible for the inactivation of epinephrine and norepinephrine. In earlier experiments, Nasmyth (1955) already found that the epinephrine-induced release of ascorbic acid from the adrenal gland is potentiated by CPZ. These results are of great interest in that they may directly relate to the observation that CPZ inhibits the uptake of exogenous norepinephrine into catecholamine storage sites (Axelrod et al., 1961 b; Hertting et al., 1961), which have to be regarded as important inactivators of the physiologic and pharmacologic effects of amines (vide III B, 4 a).

In contrast to the adrenolytic effect, the cholinolytic and antihistaminic effects of CPZ are considerably weaker than those of promethazine (Courvoisier et al., 1953; Kopera and Armitage, 1954). In this respect, other phenothiazines are more effective than CPZ. Rummel (1961) untertook a comparative study of the adrenolytic, antiserotonin and antihistaminic properties of phenothiazines on the isolated terminal ileum of guinea pig and reported the relative activity of the compounds. Courvoisier et al. (1957 d) attempted to correlate the intensity of the *in vitro* antiserotonin activity of phenothiazines with their central "sedative" effect. This attempt was apparently influenced by the hypothesis of Wooley and Shaw (1957) and of Gaddum (1957) who postulated that brain 5-HT plays an important role in the etiology of psychoses. Subsequently, this hypothesis became less tenable (vide III C, 1 a α), and all experiments designed to detect a correlation of the peripheral adrenolytic and anti-5HT effects with the central effects of CPZ observed in psychoses failed to bring forth useful results.

Table 1. *Inhibition of the effects of acetylcholine, nicotine, epinephrine, histamine, relative potency ratios;*

	pro-methazine	pro-mazine	metho-promazine	ace-promazine	fluo-promazine	tri-meprazine	levo-mepromazine
Anti-acetyl-choline (isol. ileum)	6.6 [22]	0.36 [22]	—	0.36 [22]	1 [19]	3 [8]	~ 1 [9]
Anti-nicotine (isol. ileum)	10 [22]	1.8 [22]	—	2.5 [22]	—	—	—
Anti-epinephrine — seminal vesicle	—	0.14 [22]	—	100 [22]	—	—	—
Anti-epinephrine — toxicity	—	0.2 [22]	~ 1 [5]	4 [22]	—	0.25 [8]	—
Anti-epinephrine — nictitating membrane	—	0.2 [22]	—	4 [22]	—	—	—
Anti-histamine — isol. ileum	—	—	—	—	1 [19]	10 [8]	—
Anti-histamine — bronchial constrict. in vivo	> 40 [8] 15 [22] 1.5 [25]	3 [22]	—	1 [22]	—	> 40 [8] 16 [24]	40 [9]
Anti-5-HT	~ 0.1 [24]	—	—	—	1 [19]	~ 1 [24]	5 [9]
Anti-BaCl$_2$	7 [22]	0.53 [22]	—	0.36 [22]	—	—	—

[22] Wirth et al. (1959).
[23] Haley et al. (1960).
[24] Schmid et al. (1959).

2. Effects on Heart, Circulation and Vasculature

Phenothiazines possess distinct effects on the cardiovascular system. Thus CPZ has an antifibrillatory, quinidine-like action on isolated rabbit atria (Ryall, 1956). In the Langendorff isolated rabbit heart preparation CPZ (0.05—1.0 mg) increases coronary flow. However, promethazine is more potent in this respect (Courvoisier et al., 1953). In many instances, a tachycardia develops after CPZ injection, and the epinephrine-induced increase in heart rate is not antagonized (Jourdan et al., 1955). CPZ, injected intravenously, lowers blood pressure in many species (Courvoisier et al., 1953; Huidobro, 1954; Kopera and Armitage, 1954, among others). In

5-HT and bariumchloride by phenothiazine derivatives. (The numbers express the chlorpromazine = 1)

mepazine	thio-ridazine	perazine	pro-chlorperazine	tri-fluoperazine	per-phenazine	flu-phenazine	thio-propazate	chlor-prothixene
—	2.3 [23]	0.36 [22]	0.2 [22] 2 [13]	—	~1 [4]	—	—	6.4 [21]
—	—	1.4 [22]	1.1 [22]	—	—	—	—	—
—	—	0.03 [22]	0.05 [22]	—	—	—	—	—
—	<1 [23]	0.09	0.04 [22] 0.17 [13]	—	—	—	—	—
—	—	0.2 [22]	0.4 [22]	—	—	—	—	—
	0.7 [23]				0.4 [15] ~1 [4]			0.3 [21]
—	—	2 [22]	0.5 [22]	—	—	—	—	—
—	9.1 [23]	—	0.5 [13]	—	~1 [4]	—	—	—
—	—	0.27 [22]	0.21 [22] 1—2 [13]	—	~1 [4]	—	0.3 [16]	3 [21]

man, orthostatic hypotension and even collapse after high doses occur, probably as a consequence of blockade of vascular reflex regulating mechanisms. However, spontaneous tolerance develops during prolonged treatment. The finding that intravenous injection of CPZ prevents the hypotension and bradycardia in response to electrical stimulation of the peripheral end of the cut vagus nerve can be explained by an "atropine-like" blockade of the acetylcholine effect. On the other hand, the CPZ-induced blockade of the vasopressor effect in response to carotid occlusion or electrical stimulation of the central stump of the vagal nerve is due to an adrenergic blocking effect. Peripheral vascular resistance diminishes and the peripheral vessels dilate. This is evident from the results of Courvoisier et al. (1953) who observed that a concentration of 0.1—1 mg/ml of CPZ in the perfusion fluid increases blood flow through a rabbit ear by 50—100%. CPZ inhibits the vasoconstriction in response to exogenous epinephrine (Kopera and Armitage, 1954). According to Courvoisier et al. (1953), vascular dilation and increased capillary permeability due to application of skin irritants is prevented by CPZ although all phenothiazine derivatives *per se* have tissue irritating properties upon local application. The reduction of the rat paw edema may in part be the result of a diminution of capillary permeability by resorbed CPZ (see also Hertting and Stoklaska, 1959).

3. Muscle Relaxant Effect

The muscle relaxant effect of CPZ is noteworthy. Courvoisier et al. (1953) noticed that CPZ prolongs the curarization effect of gallamine triethiodide. Furthermore, Kopera and Armitage (1954) found that intra-arterially injected CPZ blocks the muscle contraction elicited by direct and indirect stimulation in cats. On the basis of experiments on the gastrocnemius preparation in cat and guinea pig and on the rat phrenic nerve-diaphragm, Ryall (1956) concluded that CPZ diminishes the muscle contraction by blocking neuromuscular transmission and by a direct depressing effect on the muscle. Jindal and Deshpande (1961) decribed a nicotine-like blocking effect on the end plate region induced by CPZ, prochlorperazine and promethazine in *in vivo* experiments on dogs. Henatsch and Ingvar (1956) demonstrated a selective paralysis of the γ-fiber system by CPZ. The rapidly developing adaptation and the extrapyramidal side-effects make it impossible to utilize this property clinically (Domino, 1964).

4. Miscellaneous Effects

Small doses of CPZ stimulate respiration; large doses paralyse it (Courvoisier et al., 1953). The analeptic effects of nikethamide and amphetamine are blocked by CPZ. Contrary to the opinion of Courvoisier et al. (1953), CPZ does not seem to have ganglionic blocking properties (Huidobro, 1954). The local anesthetic effect of CPZ is pronounced (Courvoisier et al., 1953; Kopera and Armitage, 1954). The direct spasmolytic effect of CPZ is negligible (Courvoisier et al., 1953).

C. Central Effects

1. Effects on the Spinal Cord

Phenothiazines appear to have only insignificant direct effects on the spinal cord. After high spinalization, the depression of mono-synaptic reflexes, e. g. knee jerk, observed in intact cats after injection of CPZ and promazine (Silvestrini and Maffii, 1959) can no longer be produced (Hudson and Domino, 1961). Similar results are reported by Preston (1956). In animals with intact neuraxis, polysynaptic reflexes (e. g., linguomandibular reflex) are less suscep-tible to CPZ or promazine depression than the monosynaptic reflexes (Silvestrini and Maffii, 1959). Moreover, Dasgupta and Werner (1955) demonstrated that CPZ diminishes the crossed extensor reflex in the decerebrate cat to a considerably greater extent than in the spinalized preparation. It, therefore, appears that the supraspinal influence of CPZ is of great importance for its action on the spinal cord, and in this respect, Russian investigators (vide Domino, 1962 a) call particular attention to the reticular formation. Domino (1962 a) emphasizes that the effect of CPZ on the spinal cord is due mainly to an inhibition of reticular reflex activating areas in the medulla rather than the consequence of facilitation of bulbar inhibitory mechanisms.

2. Influence on Medullary, Mesencephalic and Diencephalic Autonomic Functions

The significance of the reticular formation for the effect of CPZ on the spinal cord has already been emphasized in the previous section. In this connection, it is noteworthy that decerebrate rigidity is abolished by CPZ (Henatsch and Ingvar, 1956).

a) Antiemetic Effect

The antiemetic effect of phenothiazine derivatives is due to their action on the chemoreceptor trigger zone as evidenced by the marked inhibition of apomorphine emesis in dogs (Courvoisier et al., 1953), whereas copper sulfate-induced vomiting can not be prevented by CPZ. According to Schallek et al. (1956), doses of 0.1 mg/kg s. c. of CPZ are sufficient to prevent apomorphine emesis in dogs. It is, however, interesting that phenothiazine derivatives exert no anti-emetic effect in cats (Jacobsen, 1959). There is no doubt about the

9

Table 2. *Inhibition of apomorphine-emesis and the*
(Significance of

	pro-methazine	pro-mazine	metho-promazine	ace-promazine	fluo-promazine	tri-meprazine	levo-mepromazine
Anti-apomorphine effect: dog	—	<1 [18]	1 [5]	1 [18]	10 [19]	0.3 [8]	1 [9]
pigeon	—	0.1 [29]	—	—	4.4 [29]	—	—
Hypothermic effect	—	7 [18] 0.5 [6]	—	<1 [18] 0.8 [6]	—	0.7 [8]	1.7 [9] 0.7 [6]

[27] Rosenkilde and Govier (1957).
[28] Wang (1958).
[29] Burkman (1962).

antiemetic effect of phenothiazines in man with the exception of thioridazine which is supposedly devoid of antiemetic properties. Motion sickness is not ameliorated by phenothiazines, in spite of the fact that CPZ antagonizes vomiting induced in dogs by rotation (Cook and Toner, 1954). The antiemetic effectiveness of various phenothiazines does not parallel other central effects of these agents (Courvoisier et al., 1957 d).

b) Influence on Central Mechanisms Governing Circulation

Phenothiazines inhibit the central regulatory mechanism of circulation by their effect on the medulla oblongata and on the hypothalamus. Already mentioned was the finding of Courvoisier et al. (1953) that intravenous injection of CPZ diminishes the vasopressor response to bilateral carotid occlusion and to electrical stimulation of the central portion of the cut vagus nerve. While a peripheral adrenolytic effect of CPZ cannot be excluded in these experiments, Dasgupta and Werner (1954) were able to elicit a fall in blood pressure and a diminution of the carotid sinus baroreceptor reflex by intracisternal injections of very small, peripherally presumably inactive doses of CPZ (50—100 γ/kg) in cats (see also Schmitt and Schmitt, 1961). Jourdan et al. (1955) reported that CPZ, injected into the vertebral artery, elicits a fall in blood pressure, and similar observations were made by Tangri and Bhargava (1960) after injecting CPZ into the ventricle. Furthermore, CPZ also inhibites vasopressor reflexes elicited by sciatic stimulation, carotid occlusion (Wang et al., 1964) or

thio-mepazine	ridazine	perazine	pro-chlorperazine	tri-fluoperazine	per-phenazine	flu-phenazine	thio-propazate	chlor-prothixene
—	—	2 [18]	3.0 [27] 4 [13]	—	24 [27] 17—48 [28]	34—124 [29]	4.6 [16]	1 [21]
—	—	—	2.3 [29]	7.2 [29]	10.2 [29]	27 [29]	—	—
0.1 [6]	0.4 [13] 0.1 [10] 0.4 [11]	0.3 [18]	0.4 [13] 0.6 [6]	0.4 [6]	0.4 [6]	—	0.6 [16]	1.3 [6]

direct electrical stimulation of the vasomotor medullary centers in the isolated perfused head of dogs. Wang et al. (1964) called attention to the finding that in some experiments, large doses of CPZ (20 mg/kg) reverse the inhibition of the vasomotor medullary centers induced by small doses of CPZ (0.1 mg/kg). In this connection, the experiments of Martin et al. (1960) and Schmitt and Schmitt (1961) are of interest. They demonstrated that the vasopressor effect of intravenously injected NE is diminished by small doses of CPZ and enhanced by large doses.

c) Effects on Body Temperature

Most phenothiazines lower body temperature, particularly in a low temperature environment. This effect was described for CPZ by Courvoisier et al. (1953). The hypothermia appears to be due to an inhibition of hypothalamic regulatory centers, though a concomitant effect on peripheral vasculature may also play a role (see this chapter B, 2). Again, this hypothermic effect of phenothiazines does not parallel other central actions (e. g., the antiemetic effect) (Courvoisier et al., 1957 d).

Hyperthermia produced by pyrogens is also antagonized by CPZ (Courvoisier et al., 1953; Cheymol and Levassort, 1955). However, it is doubtful whether CPZ, on the basis of these findings, can be classified as an antipyretic (Brendel and L'Allemand, 1955). An extensive discussion of this question can be found in the review by Eichler-Satke (1958). Phenothiazines, due to their hypothermic effect, may affect some of the temperature-dependent biochemical mechanisms (vide this chapter C, 5, c).

d) Effect on Appetite

Clinical experience shows that phenothiazines stimulate appetite, often resulting in considerable gain of body weight. The increased appetite may be due to inhibition of certain hypothalamic centers. Under certain conditions, this may make chronic therapy with phenothiazines unfeasible.

e) Influence on Central Sympathetic Mechanisms

In cats, morphine causes a stimulation of "sympathetic centers" resulting in hyperirritability, catecholamine release from the adrenal medulla and a diminution of NE concentration in the hypothalamus (Holzbauer and Vogt, 1954). Although CPZ (see this chapter, C7c, β) prevents the morphine-induced stimulation, it does not influence the biochemical events accompanying the excitation of hypothalamic sympathetic centers. In addition, the ascorbic acid depletion induced by stressing rats can not be prevented by CPZ (Holzbauer and Vogt, 1954); this is in contrast to the positive results reported by Mafouz and Ezz (1958).

Minimal external stimuli elicit a maximal sympathetic excitation of central and peripheral nature in decerebrate cats. This so-called "sham-rage" is characterized by rage (hissing and clawing), piloerection, maximal dilatation of pupils, retraction of the nictitating membrane and other signs of sympathetic stimulation. Dasgupta et al. (1954) demonstrated that the "sham-rage" reaction is blocked by small doses of CPZ (0.25 mg/kg i. v.). This dose of CPZ is too small to have a significant peripheral adrenolytic effect. It is therefore assumed that CPZ inhibits those central sympathetic mechanisms which are involved in the "sham-rage" reaction.

The phenothiazine derivatives have numerous centrally mediated effects on the function of endocrine glands, possibly through their action on the hypothalamus. These effects will be discussed in this chapter, section D.

3. Influence on Bioelectrical Phenomena in the CNS

The vast literature on the effects of phenothiazines on electrophysiological phenomena in the brain makes it impossible to discuss at length even the more important publications. The reader, who desires complete information on this subject, is referred to competent reviews (Killam, 1962; Domino, 1962 a; Bradley, 1963).

a) Changes in the EEG

CPZ and other phenothiazine derivatives synchronize the normal EEG pattern. This effect was first described in man in 1952 by Terzian. From the many subsequent investigations on the EEG-effects of CPZ, it can be stated that small doses of CPZ cause an enhancement of α-activity, whereas after large doses, bursts of δ-waves appear and eventually become dominant. However, spindles, as they occur during normal sleep, are absent. It should be emphasized that these EEG changes are not seen in every case. Clinically active doses of CPZ do not appear to be able to suppress the EEG desynchronisation induced by external stimuli (Shagass, 1955).

The EEG synchronizing effect of CPZ is observed in many animal species. This effect was first described by Terzian (1954) in rabbits and by Hiebel et al. (1954) in dogs and cats immobilized with gallamine triethiodide. Many other authors have essentially confirmed this finding and extended the observation to other species (Longo et al., 1954; Das et al., 1954; Rinaldi and Himwich, 1955 a; Gangloff and Monnier, 1957; Longo, 1960). Rabbits are particularly sensitive and readily respond to CPZ with synchronization of the EEG. However, large sublethal doses of CPZ desynchronize the rabbit EEG (Rinaldi and Himwich, 1955 a). In cats contradictory results have been obtained. Thus, Bradley and Hance (1957) observed an EEG synchronizing effect in animals with chronically implanted electrodes, whereas Killam et al. (1957) could not show any significant changes with doses of 2—6 mg/kg of CPZ. Bradley and Hance (1957), and Martin et al. (1958) found evidence of cortical synchronization in the cat encéphale isolé preparation. In contrast, CPZ does not alter the EEG activity in the cerveau isolé preparation of the cat (Bradley and Hance, 1957) nor of the isolated cerebral cortex of the dog (Preston, 1956). These results make it unlikely that the EEG changes after administration of CPZ are due to a direct effect on these brain areas.

b) Effect on EEG Arousal Reaction

The EEG arousal reaction resulting in a desynchronization of the electrocorticogram can be elicited either by stimulation of various peripheral afferent inputs or by direct electrical stimulation of the mesencephalic ascending reticular system. Various sensory stimuli (osmotic, acoustic, optic, tactile, pain), afferent nerve stimulation and "humoral" stimulation (intravenous epinephrine injections) may serve as activators. All these peripheral stimuli activate the brainstem reticular formation and generate an EEG arousal reaction similar to that induced by direct stimulation of the reticular system.

There is no agreement in the literature as to the effect of CPZ on the EEG arousal reaction elicited by direct and indirect stimulation of the reticular formation. The original observation of Hiebel et al. (1954), that CPZ in small doses (2 mg/kg i. v.) prevents the EEG arousal induced by afferent stimulation and intravenous epinephrine injection, has been confirmed in experiments on cats (e. g., Martin et al., 1958; Bradley and Hance, 1957; Tokizane et al., 1957) and rabbits (Longo et al., 1954; Rinaldi and Himwich, 1955 a; Gangloff and Monnier, 1957). In contrast, Killam and Killam (1957) noted only a very weak depressing effect of CPZ on the arousal reaction evoked by electrical stimulation of the sciatic nerve in the cat. However, in rabbits there appears to be a good correlation between the suppressing effect of phenothiazines on the EEG arousal reaction and clinical usefulness. This conclusion was reached by Himwich et al. (1956) after systematic investigations and is shared by Brücke and Stumpf on the basis of an unpublished study on some 200 compounds.

The duration of EEG arousal induced by direct stimulation of the brainstem reticular formation is generally shortened by CPZ in the cat (Hiebel et al., 1954; Martin et al., 1958) and rabbit (Longo et al., 1954; Rinaldi and Himwich, 1955 a; Brücke et al., 1957; Gangloff and Monnier, 1957). Complete inhibition is observed only after large doses of CPZ. The threshold for arousal is either not significantly altered by CPZ or slightly increased. In this respect, barbiturates are far more active (Preston, 1956; Bradley and Key, 1959; Killam and Killam, 1957). It is therefore questionable if the weak direct depressant effect of phenothiazines on the brainstem arousal mechanism can serve as an explanation for their central action. In this connection, it is noteworthy that, according to Killam (1957), CPZ (1 mg/kg i. v.) enhances the inhibitory effect of the reticular formation on acoustically evoked potentials in the cochlear nucleus and in the medial geniculate body (compare this chapter, C, 3g).

c) Influence on the Electrical Activity of the Reticular Formation

Spontaneous discharge rates of those neurons in the reticular formation which show convergence are reduced by 2—4 mg/kg i. v. of CPZ. The response of these neurons to sensory stimulation, in particular to physiological input, is also diminished (Bradley, 1963). According to De Maar et al. (1958), potentials evoked in the reticular formation by sciatic stimulation in the cat are increased by 10 to 15 mg/kg of CPZ (see also Killam and Killam, 1959). The amplitude of both short and long latency potentials is enhanced, and the absolute refractory period of the latter is prolonged. Pentobarbital, on the other hand, decreases these potentials and prolongs the refractory period of the short latency responses.

d) Influence on the Thalamic Projection System

The specific relay nuclei of the thalamus are not significantly influenced by CPZ (Preston, 1956; Killam, 1957; Killam and Killam, 1959). The excitability of the ventro-lateral thalamic nucleus is somewhat enhanced in the unanesthetized rabbit (Monnier and Krupp, 1959), and stimulation of the lateral thalamus lowers the threshold for after-discharges and prolongs them (Gangloff and Monnier, 1957). In monkeys with chronically implanted electrodes, CPZ slightly raises the threshold for behavioral arousal elicited by stimulation of the nucleus ventralis posterior (Takaori and Deneau, 1962 a).

The diffuse thalamic projection system is barely depressed by CPZ as evidenced by the thalamo-cortical recruiting responses; these are only slightly diminished by 2 mg/kg of CPZ (Killam and Killam, 1956; Dasgupta et al., 1954). In the unanesthetized rabbit, Gangloff and Monnier (1957) found that the threshold for the thalamo-cortical recruiting response is lowered after injection of 5 mg/kg CPZ intravenously. The threshold for the EEG and behavioral arousal elicited by high frequency stimulation of the diffuse thalamic projection system is only slightly increased by 4—6 mg/kg CPZ (Killam et al., 1957).

e) Effect on the Limbic System

EEG arousal in the hippocampus of the rabbit (theta rhythm) is depressed by CPZ and other phenothiazines but to a lesser extent than in the cortex (Brücke et al., 1957 b).

The phenothiazines appear to have numerous direct effects on the limbic system. Preston (1956) found that large doses of CPZ (20 mg/kg) elicit seizure discharges in the hippocampus, and particularly in the amygdaloid nuclei. Extremely large doses (40 mg/kg) cause spreading of the spikes to the cortex. According to Killam et al.

15

(1957), CPZ in small doses (5 mg/kg) shortens the generalized clonic phase of rhinencephalic paroxysms in cats induced by electrical stimulation of the nuclei amygdalae and hippocampus. The rhinencephalic component itself is not changed. On the other hand, if the rhinencephalic seizures are evoked by stimulation of the afferent fibers of the fornix, CPZ inhibits the rhinencephalic component of the spike potentials (Killam and Killam, 1957). In rabbits, Monnier and Krupp (1959) found only a slight depressant effect of CPZ on convulsive discharges in response to hippocampal stimulation. In monkeys, similarly weak depressant effects of CPZ on the bioelectrical potentials of the limbic system were noted (Delgado and Mihailovic, 1956; Takaori and Deneau, 1962 a).

Interesting, though not easy to interpret, are some results of Adey and Dunlop (1960). These authors investigated neuronal discharges in the caudate nucleus and globus pallidus in response to sciatic and amygdaloid stimulation. Normally the discharge rate of pallidal neurons is not altered, or, at most, only slightly reduced in response to sciatic stimulation, but after injection of 2 mg/kg of CPZ i. v. it was clearly increased. The same result was obtained by stimulating the amygdaloid nucleus, and the effect was even more pronounced by simultaneous sciatic and amygdaloid stimulation.

f) Effects on the Cortex

Phenothiazines seem to have only very weak direct effects on the cortex. In monkeys, the threshold for eliciting motor reactions is not influenced (Delgado and Mihailovic, 1956) or only slightly increased (Takaori and Deneau, 1962 a) by CPZ. As already mentioned, CPZ, even in large doses (50 mg/kg i. v.), has no effect on the isolated hemisphere preparation in the cat (Preston, 1956). Dasgupta and Werner (1955), on the other hand, found that CPZ inhibits motor responses elicited by stimulation of the area cruciata of the cortex. The transcallosal response is not affected by CPZ (Marrazzi, 1957). However, the diminution of the transcallosal response induced by epinephrine, 5-HT, mescaline and LSD can be prevented by CPZ (Marrazzi, 1957). This effect is claimed to parallel the clinical efficacy of phenothiazine derivatives. In unanesthetized rabbits, 5—10 mg/kg of CPZ increases the threshold for cortical after-discharges evoked by stimulation of the sensory motor cortex. Interestingly, the duration of after-discharges is prolonged (Gangloff and Monnier, 1957). Unna and Martin (1957) observed an increase in cortical potentials in reponse to sciatic stimulation after i. v. injection of CPZ (5 mg/kg) in cats.

g) Interpretation of the Electrophysiological Effects

There is almost universal agreement that the "electrophysiologic" locus of action of the phenothiazine derivatives is in the brainstem reticular formation including the hypothalamus and the diffuse thalamic projection system. There is also an important direct influence of phenothiazine derivatives on the limbic system (Preston, 1956) which is anatomically and functionally connected to the reticular system. The mechanism of action of phenothiazines on the reticular formation is, however, rather hypothetical. Many authors, including Terzian (1954), assume that these agents exert a direct effect on those mechanisms of the reticular formation which are responsible for the arousal reaction (e. g., Longo et al., 1954; Hiebel et al., 1954; Rinaldi and Himwich, 1955 a; Dasgupta, 1962). Bradley (1963) modified this hypothesis, postulating that phenothiazine derivatives primarily block afferent impulses in the sensory collateral fibers to the brainstem. Killam (1962), on the basis of her own observations and the results of De Maar et al., (1958), believes that phenothiazines have no direct depressant effect on the reticular formation but facilitate inhibitory "filtering" mechanisms, thereby leading to a reduction of stimuli reaching the cortex. De Maar et al. (1958) expressed the view that the depressant effect of phenothiazines on the arousal mechanism is effected through inhibition of long latency, slow conducting pathways in the reticular formation.

The large number of hypotheses on the "electrophysiological" mechanism of action of phenothiazine derivatives in brain may be confusing but can be understood if one considers that most investigators have conducted their experiments only in one species and under special conditions. It is known that species differences greatly affect electrophysiological results. The multitude of hypotheses also demonstrates that it is impossible to characterize the mechanism of action of these agents on brain by electrophysiological experiments alone.

4. Results from Behavioral Investigations

a) Influence on General Behavior

CPZ and other phenothiazines in doses which have no significant sedative effect reduce motor activity in animals. The exploratory behavior (e. g., of the rat) is markedly diminished. The animals have no interest in food, and their reactivity to external stimuli is often reduced.

Normally aggressive rhesus monkeys are tamed by CPZ (Das et al., 1954). To differentiate the effect of centrally active agents on behavior, Norton and Beer (1956) classified the behavioral profile of cats into several categories. In this system, CPZ increases sociability and decreases hostility in cats. However, the value of this type of behavioral investigation is, as Dews and Morse (1961) comment, problematic, because it is based on a subjective method and does not allow dose-response relationships to be established.

Beside the classical observations of Delay and Deniker (1952), many investigations have been conducted on the influence of CPZ on human behavior (Heimann and Witt, 1955; Kornetsky, 1960), often utilizing batteries of psychological tests. In one comparative study, an unexpected finding was that CPZ had a greater hypnogenic effect than the same dose of secobarbital (Kornetsky and Humphries, 1958); the performance in psychological tests was not as good as before administration of the compounds, and the after-effects were equally pronounced after administration of both agents.

b) Effect on Operant Conditioned Behavior

A simple type of a conditioned response can be elicited when an animal is trained to respond to the presentation of a visual or auditory stimulus in order to avoid an unpleasant situation, e. g., a rat is trained to respond to a tone (conditioning stimulus) by jumping onto a pole (avoidance response) thus avoiding electric shock (unconditioned stimulus) which follows the tone. A flight reaction occurring only after presentation of the electric shock is called escape response. There are numerous modifications of this simple procedure. Certain behavior can be reinforced with food. Animals can also learn to avoid punishment by suppressing certain behavior. Furthermore, centrally active agents may be studied on animals exposed to conflict situations.

The interpretation of results obtained by operant conditioning techniques is at present extremely difficult since it is not apparent which central mechanisms influencing animal behavior are altered. It is also difficult to correlate behavioral phenomena with electro-physiologic and biochemical data. Moreover, it is uncertain if there is a connection between the effect of phenothiazines on conditioned behavior in animals and the antipsychotic action of these agents in man. For these reasons, it is justifiable to forego an extensive description of the numerous studies made with phenothiazines in this area. Reference is made to the competent reviews by Dews and Morse (1961), and Cook and Kelleher (1962).

Courvoisier et al. (1953) first demonstrated that CPZ (1 mg/kg s. c.) selectively blocks the conditioned avoidance response in rats. In contrast, phenobarbital in comparable doses blocks both the conditioned and unconditioned (escape) response (Cook and Weidley, 1957). Gatti (1957) was able to influence the avoidance response with doses as small as 0.1 mg/kg of CPZ. The observations of Courvoisier et al. (1953) have subsequently been confirmed many times and in species other than the rat (dogs, cats, monkeys), sometimes by means of very complex conditioning procedures. In man, similar effects have been observed with CPZ, prochlorperazine, methoxyphenothiazine and mepazine (Alexander and Horner, 1961; Windsor, 1957). The interpretation of animal experiments is particularly difficult since CPZ inhibits not only negatively motivated behavior (anxiety), but also positively motivated behavior (reward) (see Taeschler and Loew, 1965).

The method introduced by Olds (1958) rests on a different principle involving the investigation of behavioral output evoked by self-stimulation of the brain. Rats are trained to stimulate their own brains through chronically implanted electrodes by pressing a lever. It was found that the self-stimulation rate is particularly high when the electrodes are located in certain areas of the mesencephalon and diencephalon (reward area). CPZ reduces the self-stimulation rate elicited in the ventral thalamus or in the amygdaloid complex. The depressant influence of CPZ on septal self-stimulation is less evident (Olds et al., 1956, 1957). In spite of these ingenious and novel procedures, it is not possible at present to explain the results obtained with this method.

The investigations of Taeschler and Cerletti (1959) are of particular note. These authors attempted to correlate the psychological and motor behavior of animals with clinical effectiveness of phenothiazine derivatives. It was concluded that the inhibitory effect of several phenothiazines (CPZ, perphenazine, thioridazine, prochlorperazine, thiopropazate) on the conditioned avoidance response correlates well with the cataleptic effect and locomotor depression in animals and with the extrapyramidal side-effects in man. On the other hand, inhibition of emotional behavior as tested by emotionally-induced defecation is

	pro-methazine	pro-mazine	metho-promazine	ace-promazine	fluo-promazine	tri-meprazine	levo-mepromazine
Inhibition of spontaneous locomotor activity	0.045 [1] 0.05 [2] < 0.01 [3]	0.3 [3] 0.4 [4] 0.23 [1]	1 [5]	0.6 [3] 12 [6]	5 [7]	~ 1 [8]	2.5 [9]
Inhibition of conditioned avoidance response	0.12 [17]	0.3 [18] 0.6 [17]	1 [5]	1 [18]	2.7 [19] 3.7 [20]	~ 0.7 [8]	1.6 [9]
Inhibition of emotional behavior	—	—	—	—	—	—	—

[1] Tedeschi et al. (1958).
[2] Fellows and Cook (1957).
[3] Sandberg (1959).
[4] Arragoni-Martelli and Kramer (1959).
[5] Courvoisier et al. (1957 b).
[6] Møller-Nielsen et al. (1962).
[7] Burke et al. (1957).
[8] Courvoisier et al. (1958).
[9] Courvoisier et al. (1957 c).
[10] Taeschler and Cerletti (1958).
[11] Swinyard et al. (1959).

largely independent of these criteria. Thus, thioridazine inhibits defecation to a greater extent than the conditioned avoidance response, whereas the reverse is true for perphenazine and thiopropazate. CPZ and prochlorperazine exert equally marked effects in both tests. This bears some relation to the therapeutic and extrapyramidal effects of these agents in man. The clinically observed neuroleptic activity is therefore not adequately reflected in animal tests such as the conditioned avoidance escape response, locomotor activity and induced catalepsy, but rather correlates with the inhibition of emotional behavior in animals.

5. Biochemical Effects on the CNS

Phenothiazine and its derivatives are, from a chemical point of view, lipid soluble, surface active agents of great potential reactivity. Therefore, it must be expected that they influence many biochemical systems *in vitro* and *in vivo*.

a) Influence on Respiration, Oxidative Phosphorylation, Phospholipid Metabolism and Various Enzymes

The influence of phenothiazine derivatives on respiration, oxidative phosphorylation, on the activity of various enzymes and

escape response, emotional behavior by phenothiazine derivatives.
numbers, see Table 1)

mepazine	thio-ridazine	perazine	prochlor-perazine	tri-fluoperazine	per-phenazine	flu-phenazine	thio-propazate	chlor-prothixene
0.04[3]	0.26[10]		1.9[12]	6.3[14]	8.4[15]		10[16]	
			0.8[1]	1.6[6]	13[4]	—		6[6]
0.03[1]	1[11]		1[13]		21[3]		7.3[12]	

mepazine	thio-ridazine	perazine	prochlor-perazine	tri-fluoperazine	per-phenazine	flu-phenazine	thio-propazate	chlor-prothixene
1[20]	0.13[12]				13.7[15]		10[16]	
		~0.3[18]	2.4[12]	10[14]	10[14]	—		~1[21]
0.3[17]	0.8[20]				11[12]		8[12]	

mepazine	thio-ridazine	perazine	prochlor-perazine	tri-fluoperazine	per-phenazine	flu-phenazine	thio-propazate	chlor-prothixene
—	6.6[12]	—	2.9[12]	—	4.3[12]	—	5.1[12]	—

[12] Taeschler et al. (1960).　　　　[17] Desci (1961).
[13] Courvoisier et al. (1957 d).　　[18] Wirth et al. (1958).
[14] Tedeschi et al. (1959 a).　　　[19] Piala et al. (1959).
[15] Roth et al. (1959).　　　　　[20] Bhargava and Chandra (1964).
[16] Stone et al. (1960).　　　　　[21] Møller-Nielsen and Neuhold (1959).

enzyme systems and on phospholipid metabolism in the brain has been recently summarized by Richter (1961), Domino (1962 b) and Bain and Mayer (1962).

From the numerous experimental data, the following can be summarized: the inhibitory effect of CPZ and other phenothiazines on enzyme systems containing the prosthetic group, flavin adenine dinucleotide (FAD), appears to be rather specific (Helper et al., 1958; Dawkins et al., 1959). CPZ seems to behave like a true flavin antagonist (Löw, 1959; see also Yagi et al., 1956), and FAD is claimed to antagonize the EEG effects of CPZ (Yagi et al., 1960). This enzyme-inhibiting effect of phenothiazines, coupled with the property of decreasing cell membrane permeability (Spirtes and Guth, 1961, 1963; Freemann and Spirtes, 1963; Seeman and Bialy, 1963), could possibly explain the effect on the respiratory enzymes and the uncoupling of oxidative phosphorylation by these agents (Richter, 1961, and Domino, 1962 b). The inhibition of normal tissue respiration by large doses of CPZ (10^{-2} molar) (Courvoisier et al., 1953) and the inhibition of respiration in brain slices stimulated by potassium ions (Quastel, 1959) or electrical stimulation (McIlwain and Greengard, 1957) can be explained by the same mechanism. However, it remains doubtful if the very specific pharmacologic and clinical effects of these drugs on the CNS are in any way causally related to the biochemical effects, many of which are operative only *in vitro*. Thus Grenell et al. (1955) could not find evidence for uncoupling of oxidative phosphorylation in rat brain *in vivo* by CPZ. Other effects are only obtained in doses far in excess of the usual pharmacological and clinical doses. It is therefore significant that phenothiazines, in doses which are close to those used clinically, markedly influence the phospholipid metabolism of brain *in vitro* as well as *in vivo* (Rossiter, 1957; Richter, 1961; Domino, 1962 b). The practical significance of these effects is at present difficult to evaluate since some data still appear to be contradictory.

Desci's (1961) finding that there is a good correlation between *in vivo* uncoupling of phosphorylation, inhibition of conditioned reflexes and prolongation of hexobarbital sleeping time induced by phenothiazines, is undoubtedly interesting, but the practical significance must be regarded as uncertain. This is clearly evident from the observations of Taeschler et al. (1960) who found no correlation between the effect of phenothiazines on conditioned reflexes, duration of sleeping time and clinical usefulness. Seeman and Bialy (1963), on the other hand, noticed a relationship between the ability of phenothiazines to lower surface tension and their clinical usefulness.

Of more immediate significance are the biochemical effects of phenothiazines on the metabolism of endogenous transmitter substances in the brain. These effects will therefore be discussed in more detail.

b) Acetylcholine Metabolism

Dobkin et al. (1954) reported that CPZ inhibits the liberation of acetylcholine in cat brain. Similar results were obtained by the same authors using human cortical tissue obtained during lobotomy of schizophrenic patients. These observations are of interest in connection with the finding of Whittaker (1961) that CPZ in concentrations of 10^{-5} molar stabilizes the acetylcholine-containing synaptic vesicles of nerve tissue by incubation *in vitro*. It is not known if this effect is specific for phenothiazine derivatives or if it only represents the membrane stabilizing effects of these agents (Spirtes and Guth, 1961, 1963). Toman (1963) raises the question of whether this membrane stabilization could not simply be due to protein denaturation which would be sufficient to prevent all osmotic processes.

c) Norepinephrine, Dopamine and 5-HT Metabolism

A large body of information exists on the influence of phenothiazines on norepinephrine, dopamine and 5-HT in brain. The concentration of these amines in brain is not altered by CPZ (Brodie et al.,
1956 b; Vogt, 1957; Holzer and Hornykiewicz, 1959; Starbuck and
Heim, 1959; Pletscher and Gey, 1959, 1960; Ehringer et al., 1960;
Gey and Pletscher, 1961 a). This does not imply that CPZ has no
effect on amine metabolism since Cammanni et al. (1959) found that
CPZ blocks the preventive action of the monoamine oxidase (MAO)-
inhibitor, iproniazid, against reserpine-induced catecholamine release
from the adrenal. This finding was corroborated in studies on rat brain
(Ehringer et al., 1960; Pletscher and Gey, 1960). It was also reported
that CPZ prevents the iproniazid-induced increase of norepinephrine
(Pletscher and Gay, 1960) and 5-HT (Bartlet, 1960; Ehringer et al.,
1960; Pletscher and Gay, 1960) in rat brain, whereas the rise in
dopamine concentration is unaffected (Gey and Pletscher, 1961 a, b).
This iproniazide blocking effect is also seen with chlorprothixine (Gey
and Pletscher, 1961 a, b). Reserpine-induced 5-HT release from rat
brain is also diminished by CPZ. This reserpine-CPZ antagonism is,
however, only detectable during the first few hours of reserpine action
(Pletscher and Gey, 1960) and can not be demonstrated 16 hours later
(Ehringer et al., 1960). Furthermore, CPZ reduces the increase of
5-HT after *in vivo* injection of 5-hydroxytryptophane (Gey and
Pletscher, 1961 a; 1962 a). Schanberg and Giarman (1962) found that
CPZ increase the free brain 5-HT not bound to subcellular particles.

This series of results demonstrates that CPZ and probably other
phenothiazines affect amine metabolism in brain. The effects of CPZ
can not be explained by inhibition of MAO (Ehringer et al., 1960),
DOPA (3,4-dihydroxyphenylalanine) or 5-HTP (5-hydroxytrypto-
phan)-decarboxylase (Gey et al., 1961). Nevertheless, Hornykiewicz
et al. (1961) pointed out that some of these *in vivo* effects of CPZ may
be due to hypothermia since they can be prevented if the animals are
maintained at elevated room temperatures (see Pletscher and Da Prada,
1967).

It is likely that there is a relationship between the above results
obtained with pharmacologically feasible doses of CPZ and *in vitro*
data indicating inhibition of catecholamine and 5-HT uptake into
cells and particles (e. g., platelets, granules of adrenal medulla brain
slices; see Gey and Pletscher, 1964). However, it should be remem-

bered that a non-specific membrane stabilizing effect of CPZ may play a role in *in vitro* experiments.

Additional information on brain catecholamine metabolism with therapeutic doses of CPZ has been obtained by measuring the metabolic products after injection of D,L-2^{14}C-dihydroxyphenylalanine (DOPA) (Gey and Pletscher, 1964). CPZ increases the concentration of the ^{14}C-phenolcarboxylic acids and decreases the ^{14}C-monoamine fraction. This indicates that CPZ accelerates the enzymatic breakdown of catecholamines, particularly NE, derived from DOPA. Axelrod et al. (1961 b) and Hertting et al. (1961) had previously demonstrated that CPZ increases the turnover of exogenous NE and inhibits the uptake into peripheral storage sites (see also Martin et al., 1960). Andén et al. (1964 b) measured the effect of CPZ on endogenous levels of phenocarboxylic acids in brain and found that their concentration increases independent of the hypothermia (see also Bernheimer and Hornykiewicz, 1965). Following treatment with MAO-inhibitors, catecholamine metabolites (3-methoxytyramine and normetanephrine) are also increased after injection of CPZ (5 mg/kg) and haloperidol (0.5 mg/kg), whereas no change in metabolites occurs after injection of phenoxybenzamine and promethazine (Carlsson and Lindqvist, 1963).

It is uncertain whether these changes in DOPA-metabolism are causally related to increased formation and deposition of melanin in skin occurring under the influence of solar radiation after chronic ingestion of CPZ (Satanove, 1965).

In view of the results concerning the influence of CPZ and phenothiazines on cerebral amine metabolism, the following hypothesis can be developed: On the basis of electrophysiological and clinical findings (see this section, paragraphs 3 and 6), it is assumed that the principal effect of these agents is on the reticular formation, the hypo-

Table 4. *Phenothiazine-induced catalepsy in*
(Significance of numbers,

	pro-methazine	pro-mazine	metho-promazine	ace-promazine	fluo-promazine	tri-meprazine	levo-mepromazine
Catalepsy	—	< 1 [18]	—	< 1 [18] —	—	—	1 [9]
Neuroleptic effect [30]	—	0.3—0.5 —		—	2—3	—	0.6—0.9

[30] Haase and Jansen (1965).

24

thalamus, the nuclei of the extrapyramidal system and possibly the rhinencephalon. It is striking that these brain regions are particularly rich in NE, dopamine and 5-HT: NE in the central grey of the mesencephalon and in the hypothalamus (Vogt, 1954), dopamine in the putamen and caudate nucleus (Bertler and Rosengren, 1959) as well as in the substantia nigra and pallidum (Ehringer and Hornykiewicz, 1960; Hornykiewicz, 1963) and 5-HT in all these areas and in the limbic system (Bogdanski et al., 1957). The correlation between localization of cerebral amines and those brain areas on which CPZ acts indicates the importance of the biochemical results regarding the mechanism of action of CPZ. The existence of noradrenergic and dopaminergic mechanisms, which may be involved in impulse transmission within the reticular (Rothballer, 1959) and extrapyramidal (Hornykiewicz, 1964 b, c) systems respectively, gives additional weight to this viewpoint.

However, it must be emphasized that this hypothesis is supported only by indirect evidence. Moreover, it is still unclear whether phenothiazines exert their main effect on cerebral catecholamines by blockade of catecholamine receptors (analogous to the peripheral adrenolytic effect) (Carlsson and Lindqvist, 1963) or by inhibiting either storage of monoamines (Gey and Pletscher, 1964) or disposition of their metabolites (Andén et al., 1964 b).

6. Extrapyramidal Motor Disturbances in Man and Catalepsy in Animals

a) Extrapyramidal Motor Disturbances in Man

Chronic treatment with many phenothiazine derivatives frequently results in symptoms which resemble the parkinson syndrome (as observed in postencephalitic and idiopathic parkinsonism). These

animals and the neuroleptic effect in man
see Table 1)

mepazine	thioridazine	perazine	prochlorperazine	trifluoperazine	perphenazine	fluphenazine	thiopropazate	chlorprothixene
			2 [12]	8 [14]				
—	~ 0.1 [10]	< 1 [18]	3—4 [13]		16 [12]	—	8 [12]	—
—	0.5—0.7	0.5—0.7	~ 4	~ 10—20	10	0.6—0.9	20—40	—

symptoms may include deficiency of will power (abulia), poverty of movements (akinesia) stiffness of muscles (rigidity), mask-like expression and, in nearly every case, tremor, which may be a fine tremor of the fingers or a violent, coarse trembling.

Other consequences of chronic phenothiazine treatment are motor restlessness (akathisia), inability to remain seated (tasikinesia), oculogyric crises, trismus, spastic protrusion of tongue, torticollis, twisting movements of extremities and opisthotonus.

All these symptoms can occur early in treatment or they may appear very late. Although their appearance may seem alarming, they are most often harmless (but see this chapter, section G, 2) and can be succesfully treated with anti-parkinsonian agents.

Extrapyramidal side-effects are particularly marked during treatment with derivatives containing a methyl-piperazine side-chain (thioperazine, butyrylperazine, among others). In contrast, thioridazine, which is also used as an antipsychotic agent, causes only mild parkinson-like disturbances. However, it is to be remembered that the piperazine derivatives are used in considerably smaller doses.

The extrapyramidal motor effects of phenothiazine derivatives are of particular interest since many investigators believe that they constitute a *conditio sine qua non* for a successful therapy of schizophrenia. Gross symptoms do not seem to be a prerequisite; the occurrence of very slight disturbances, e. g., difficulty in writing, appear to be sufficient (Haase, 1955; Brune et al., 1962 a, b; Haase and Janssen, 1965). This concept is, however, not recognized by other authors (compare with Goldman, 1962 b; Cole and Clyde, 1963), and the relationship between the intensity of extrapyramidal effects and antipsychotic properties is denied.

b) Catalepsy in Animals

"Catalepsy"—a symptom induced by phenothiazines, mainly in small rodents—manifests itself as rigidity and a lack of motor activity. The animals may be placed in unnatural positions which are maintained. An enormous amount of literature exists dealing with this phenomenon, particularly in connection with the alkaloid bulbocapnine (Brücke, 1935, 1936; Zetler and Moog, 1958). A good survey of the methods of experimentally evoked catalepsy has recently been written by Stumpf (1962). Under no circumstance should the term "catatonia" be used for describing this experimentally-induced state of rigidity and akinesia in animals since it is questionable whether this condition is at all connected to the catatonic state of schizophrenia as has been assumed (DeJong and Buruk, 1930).

Phenothiazines also induce catalepsy in higher mammals such as the cat and the monkey. In these species the similarity to the iatrogenic parkinson syndrome in man is striking. In monkeys, hysteria-like dramatic hyperkinesias can also be observed. Even birds can exhibit catalepsy. In poikilotherms, CPZ has no comparable effect on the somatic system, and these animals die in flaccid paralysis. Injection of alumina paste into the head of the caudate nucleus in cats evokes a syndrome similar to that induced by CPZ (Spiegel and Szekely, 1961). It has been repeatedly debated whether or not catalepsy and parkinsonism are analogus phenomena. Taeschler et al. (1960) believe there is a parallel between the two syndromes. In favor of this view is the observation that those phenothiazines which cause the strongest parkinson-like side-effects also produce the highest degree of catalepsy in rats. Furthermore, agents which antagonize phenothiazine-induced parkinsonism in man, also antagonize the cataleptic state in animals (Zetler et al., 1960). Thus, even phenothiazines used as anti- parkinson agents (e. g., diethazine) antagonize experimental catalepsy as well. Experimental catalepsy occurs very soon after injection of phenothiazines, whereas the parkinson syndrome in man appears after a considerably longer latency. The difference seems to be mainly due to different dosage in each case. The principal difference between catalepsy and parkinsonism is the very marked akinesia occurring in catalepsy, which explains why French authors refer to the phenomena as a mixture of parkinsonism and "catatonia".

c) *Biochemical Considerations of Phenothiazine Effects on the Extrapyramidal System*

Since recent biochemical studies have shed new light on the parkinson syndrome in man, it should be feasible to use a similar approach to the problem of phenothiazine induced "parkinsonism" (see review by Curzon, 1968).

Montagu (1957) and later, Carlsson et al. (1958) and Schümann (1959), demonstrated that the brain contains dopamine (3-hydroxy-tyramine). Bertler and Rosengren (1959) found dopamine to be specifically localized in the caudate nucleus and putamen of various animal species. This observation has been confirmed in man (Sano et al., 1959; Ehringer and Hornykiewicz, 1960; Bertler, 1961 a) and has been extended to include the substantia nigra and the external pallidum (Hornykiewicz, 1963, 1964 a).

Since 1960, Hornykiewicz and his colleagues have demonstrated in several publications that in human parkinsonism, especially of the postencephalitic type, a significant diminution of dopamine occurs in the corpus striatum (caudate nucleus and putamen) (Ehringer and Hornykiewicz, 1960; Bernheimer et al., 1963) and in the substantia nigra (Hornykiewicz, 1963). At the same time, Barbeau et al. (1961) found that parkinson patients excrete less dopamine in urine than control patients. In addition, it has been made probable that dopamine deficiency in the nuclei of the extrapyramidal system represents a biochemical change specific for the parkinson syndrome (vide Hornykiewicz, 1966 a). In experiments in which the dopamine content of extrapyramidal centers was increased by administration of DOPA, the parkinson akinesia (Birkmayer and Hornykiewicz, 1961, 1962, 1964) and parkinson rigidity (Barbeau et al., 1962) were significantly ameliorated. This led to the conclusion that akinesia is causally linked to the dopamine deficiency in the corpus striatum (for additional literature reference on the influence of DOPA on the parkinson syndrome, see chapter III, section C, 6 b). As to the mechanism of phenothiazine parkinsonism, it is possible that phenothiazines (see this chapter, section C, 5 c) influence catecholamine metabolism either by inhibiting uptake of newly formed amines into storage sites or by blocking amine receptors. In this respect, it would be of great practical significance to uncover a correlation between potency of phenothiazines on the extrapyramidal system and on dopamine receptors.

A different explanation for the parkinson-inducing effect of phenothiazines has been proposed by Himwich and Rinaldi (1957). On the basis of their observation that large doses of CPZ increase the electrical activity of the ascending reticular system in the rabbit (Rinaldi and Himwich, 1955 a; see also this chapter, section C, 3 a), they assume that this hyperactivity in the ascending reticular system also occurs in man after chronic treatment with CPZ. In addition, they assume that the hyperactivity extends to the descending reticular formation, which, according to the authors, might be the cause for the uncoordinated extrapyramidal hyperactivity after administration of phenothiazines.

The viewpoint of Himwich and Rinaldi (1957) is not incompatible with the biochemical observations mentioned above. It has been described repeatedly that experimental lesions in the reticular formation (Vernier and Unna, 1954) or in the mesencephalic tegmentum (Ward et al., 1948), as well as stimulation of reticular structures (Folkerts and Spiegel, 1953), elicits parkinson-like symptoms particularly tremor in monkeys. Folkerts and Spiegel (1953) believe that these symptoms are the consequence of a loss of control in the higher centers (substantia nigra) over the reticular system mechanism. Since those regions whose destruction induces parkinsonism are identical with areas containing dopaminergic (substantia nigra) and noradrenergic (reticular formation) neurons, it is natural to postulate that functional blockade of these regions by CPZ causes parkinson-like symptoms similar to those elicited by electro-coagulation.

7. Interaction of Phenothiazines with other Centrally Acting Agents

a) General Anesthetics and Hypnotics

Courvoisier et al. (1953) were the first to describe the potentiating effect of CPZ on ether anesthesia and barbiturate sleeping time in mice and guinea pigs. Similar observations by Zipf and Alstädter (1954), Kopera and Armitage (1954) and others followed. CPZ and other phenothiazines also enhance the effect of general anesthetics in man (Laborit and Huguenard, 1952; Staehelin and Kielholz, 1953; Zettler, 1953). Moyer found that the enhancement of general anesthesia by phenothiazines varies greatly from patient to patient. CPZ increases the central effects of ethyl alcohol in animals (Graham et al., 1957) and in man (Zirkle et al., 1959; Burge, 1961).

b) Central Stimulants, Convulsants, Physostigmine

The central stimulant effects of amphetamine and methylphenidate, whether expressed behaviorally or by the EEG arousal reaction, are inhibited by CPZ (Bradley and Hance, 1957). Amphetamine toxicity in mice, particularly when kept in groups, is considerably lowered by CPZ (Lasagna and Mc Cann, 1957; Burn and Hobbs, 1957); the same applies to methylphenidate and pipradol (Bradley, 1963). The desynchronizing effect of nicotine (Longo et al., 1954) or apomorphine (Brücke et al., 1957 a) on the EEG, and the convulsant effect of nicotine (Longo et al., 1954) or cocaine (Meidinger, 1956; Bogdanski and Spector, 1957) are diminished by CPZ. In contrast, the convulsant effect of strychnine (Courvoisier et al., 1953; Tripod, et al., 1954; Schallek et al., 1956), caffeine (Meidin-

Table 5. *Inhibition of amphetamine-induced stimulation and toxicity,*
(Significance of numbers,

	pro-methazine	pro-mazine	metho-promazine	ace-promazine	fluo-promazine	tri-meprazine	levo-meprazine
Inhibition of amphetamine hyperactivity	—	—	—	—	1 [19]	—	0.5 [25]
Amphetamine detoxification	—	—	—	—	1 [19]	—	—
Potentiation of hypnosis	~ 0.2	0.3 [18] 0.5 [3]	1 [5]	~ 1 [3] > 1 [18]	—	~ 1 [8]	~ 2 [9] ~ 1 [26]
Potentiation of morphine analgesia	—	—	1 [5]	—	~ 1 [19]	0.6 [8]	1.6 [5]

[25] Leslie and Maxwell (1964).

ger, 1956) and pentylenetetrazol are not influenced by CPZ. In rabbits, CPZ reduces the frequency of the theta rhythm induced in the hippocampus by physostigmine (Brücke et al., 1958).

c) Influence on Central Effects of Morphine

α) Analgesia. Courvoisier et al. (1953) noted that morphine analgesia in mice is enhanced by CPZ. Wirth (1954) and Schneider (1954) confirmed these results, whereas Kopera and Armitage (1954) were unable to find a potentiation of the analgesic effect of morphine. Enhancement of morphine analgesia also occurs in man (Zettler, 1953; Staehelin and Kielholz, 1953; Sadove et al., 1954). Friebel and Reichle (1955) observed that CPZ *per se* possesses analgesic properties in mice. Clinically, levomepromazine in particular is claimed to have an analgesic effect.

β) Morphine-induced Central Stimulation. In cats as well as in mice, morphine causes a marked central stimulation. CPZ and other phenothiazines prevent this effect of morphine in cats (Loewe, 1956) and in mice (Kouzmanoff et al., 1958). However, the biochemical consequences of morphine-induced excitation are not altered by CPZ (see this chapter, section C, 2 e).

D. Endocrine Effects

A detailed discussion of the endocrine effects of CPZ and other phenothiazines is found in the reviews by Domino (1962 b) and Brauchitsch (1961).

mazine	thio-perazine	ridazine	pro-chlorperazine	trifluo-perazine	per-phenazine	flu-phenazine	thio-propazate	chlor-prothixene
—	0.23[10]	0.3[18]	3.6[25]	5[25]	—	—	—	—
—	0.4[11]	—	—	—	—	—	5.6[16]	~1[21]
~0.5[3]	~1[23] 3.6[10]	—	2.5[12] 0.5[13] ~1[3]	—	~1[15] 1.4[12]	—	0.4[16] 1.2[12]	~1[21]
—	—	—	~0.4[13]	—	—	—	—	>1[21]

[26] Godwey et al. (1959).

In women, large doses of phenothiazines may lead to amenorrhea (Clark and Johnson, 1960). Postponement of ovulation and menstruation by CPZ has also been observed (Whitelaw, 1956). CPZ influences the urine excretion of several hormones. Thus, the excretion of gonadotrophines, estradiol, estrone, estriol and pregnanediol is diminished. The excretion of total 17-hydroxycorticoids is also reduced, whereas 17-ketosteroid excretion is unaffected. These changes in excretion occur in non-pregnant and pregnant women as well as during the involutional period (Suzuki et al., 1956). Since CPZ diminishes gonadotrophin excretion even in pregnant women, its effect appears to be central (hypophysis) and peripheral (chorion).

Phenothiazines cause abnormal lactation in man (Hooper et al., 1961) and animals (Sulman, 1961). In rats, CPZ releases luteotropine from the adenohypophysis inducing pseudo-pregnancy (Barraclough and Sawyer, 1959). In frogs, melanocyte-stimulating hormone is liberated from the hypophysis (Scott and Nading, 1961).

Viewpoints differ in regard to phenothiazine effects on the kidney. In man, there is a predominantly diuretic effect, whereas in water-loaded rats both diuretic and anti-diuretic effects are described (see Domino, 1962 b).

Stress-induced release of ascorbic acid from adrenal cortex—apparently a central mechanism—is prevented by CPZ (Mafouz and Ezz, 1958). This result contradicts an earlier observation by Holzbauer and Vogt (1954) who found that CPZ is ineffective in rats in this respect (see also Nasmyth, 1955).

Most authors consider the endocrine effects of CPZ to be a consequence of an inhibitory influence of this agent on the hypophysis and hypothalamus.

E. Metabolic Fate of Phenothiazines

Within the framework of this presentation, it is impossible to discuss extensively this complex problem. The reader is referred to the publication by the Pharmacology Service Center (1961), in which over 100 papers are discussed. Some important publications are also discussed in Domino's (1962 b) article. The fate of phenothiazines in the animal and human organism is not precisely known: many metabolites of CPZ have been isolated in human urine (Williams and Parke, 1964). Salzman and Brodie (1956) identified in dog and man CPZ-sulfoxide as one of the metabolites. Posner (1959) called attention to the fact that CPZ does not only metabolize to the sulfoxide, but also to the demethylated sulfoxide, N-oxide, phenolic derivatives and to the corresponding glucuronides. The paper chromatogram of human urine reveals 15 different metabolic products after ingestion of CPZ or promazine. Although CPZ-sulfoxide is considerably less effective than CPZ (Moran and Butler, 1956), it is possible that some as yet unknown metabolites are more potent than the parent agent contributing to its effectiveness. The finding of Behn et al. (1956) that phenothiazines can pass the placental barrier and appear in the urine of newborns whose mothers received phenothiazines before delivery is of special interest.

Investigations of the tissue distribution of phenothiazines have given conflicting results. Thus, Christensen and Wase (1956) reported an accumulation of ^{35}S labelled CPZ in mouse brain, whereas Walkenstein and Seifter (1959) found little radioactivity in rat brain, most of the labelled material being accumulated in lung, liver, spleen and kidney. Jaramillo and Guth (1963) recently found that CPZ and prochlorperazine accumulate in dog brain in those areas which, on the basis of the electrophysiological and biochemical data mentioned earlier, represent the most likely loci of action (medulla, hypothalamus, basal ganglia, hippocampus, amygdala and mesencephalon), whereas the concentration in cerebral cortex and cerebellum was considerably smaller. Thioethylperazine, a phenothiazine derivative with potent antiemetic effects but devoid of neuroleptic activity, accumulates mainly in the cerebellum.

F. Habituation and Withdrawal

Boyd (1960) has shown that rats can develop tolerance to CPZ as a result of which acute lethal doses are well tolerated after chronic administration. Abrupt termination of treatment leads to withdrawal symptoms. The rats exhibit hyperkinesia, diarrhea and sometimes die suddenly. Those animals which survive recuperate rapidly and within 10 days most symptoms induced by chronic CPZ treatment (diminution of body weight gain, anemia and leukocytosis) have disappeared.

In man, a degree of habituation to the CPZ-induced block of cardiovascular reflexes may occur. Patients who, after administration of large doses, cannot get up without suffering an orthostatic collapse are able to do so during the course of continuing treatment. The sudden termination of prolonged treatment with large doses of phenothiazines usually leads to exacerbation of the basic disease (see Gross et al., 1961). Many authors (Brooks, 1959; Benett and Kooi, 1961; Degkwitz and Luxenburger, 1965) believe this to be a sign of withdrawal, whereas Domino (1962 b) states that there is no reason to assume that phenothiazines induce true addiction and abstinence symptoms in man.

G. Adverse Reactions and Treatment Risks

1. Suicide and Fatal Poisoning

Even after intentional or accidental ingestion of very large doses of phenothiazines, no cases of lethal outcome have been observed. Overdosage leads to very marked central nervous system depression and prolonged hypotension. Children who accidentally ingest phenothiazines exhibit mainly extrapyramidal (dystonic) symptoms. It is noteworthy that children and women are far more susceptible to the extrapyramidal effects of phenothiazines than male adults.

2. Central Nervous System

Disturbances of the extrapyramidal motor system are relatively frequent and have already been discussed (this chapter, section C, 6 a). It is, however, remarkable that there are patients who, independent of dosage, are almost completely resistant to these side-effects. It has already been mentioned that women are more susceptible than men. The majority of older patients develop a parkinson syndrome, whereas younger patients (under 40 years) exhibit almost exclusively dys-

33

kinesias (Ayd, 1961; see also Hollister, 1964). Hereditary factors also appear to be involved (Kalow, 1962). The extrapyramidal side-effects are generally reversible. However, there is an increasing number of cases being reported in which phenothiazine derivatives cause permanent dyskinesias (Uhrbrand and Faurby, 1960; Druckmann et al., 1962; Hunter et al., 1964; Degkwitz and Luxenburger, 1965 [additional references]). Grünthal and Walther-Büel (1960) reported a fatal case with dystonic disturbances of the face and neck musculature after administration of large doses of chlorperphenazine. The authors found pathologic changes in the inferior olives as the only sign of microscopically detectable damage which they believe to be causally related to the extrapyramidal symptoms. On the basis of this experience, one has to keep in mind the possibility that morphological changes of certain brain regions may be the cause of permanent (choreiform) dyskinesias induced by phenothiazines.

Although convulsions as a consequence of phenothiazine therapy are occurring less and less frequently, Hollister (1964) mentions some cases of convulsions and hypotension after combination treatment with phenothiazines and chlordiazepoxide, one case ending in death.

3. Autonomic Nervous System

Autonomic disturbances are caused by the anticholinergic and antiadrenergic effects of phenothiazine derivatives. The atropine-like effect is predominant in most agents. Consequently, the most frequent side-effects are dryness of oral mucosa, tachycardia, peculiar grey pallor of the skin, disturbances in accommodation, constipation and micturition difficulties. With predominantly adrenolytic agents a mild hypotension and general weakness may occur. More frequent complaints appear to be disturbances in ejaculation but with preservation of the ability to have erections and orgasm. Particularly at the start of phenothiazine therapy, hypotension with susceptibility to orthostatic collapse is a frequent observation. Phenothiazines may have a quinine-like effect on the heart (Hollister, 1964).

4. Striated Musculature

It must be remembered that the symptoms of myasthenia gravis are aggravated by phenothiazines (in the case of CPZ, see McQuillen et al., 1963). This is the consequence of the neuromuscular blocking effects of these agents (see this chapter, section B, 3).

5. Jaundice

The occurrence of jaundice, which at one time was a feared complication, is considerably less frequent today. This is probably due to the wider use of phenothiazine derivatives which are safer in this respect than CPZ. The icterus appears to develop as a consequence of cholestatic action. The patients usually recover spontaneously and completely. However, hypersensitivity to these agents may persist. In rare cases, a biliary cirrhosis may develop. On the basis of the assumption that CPZ-induced jaundice is caused by a thickening of bile, Dreyfuss (1958) increased fluid intake in these patients and reduced the occurrence of jaundice from 4.4% to 0.34%.

6. Agranulocytosis

Phenothiazines belong to that class of agents which most frequently cause agranulocytosis. Panhemocytophthisis is rarely noted. According to Hollister (1964), the incidence of agranulocytosis is one case in 3000—4000 patients. Almost all phenothiazine derivatives can cause this complication. The following agents have been implicated: CPZ, promazine, mepazine, perphenazine, prochlorperazine, trifluperazine, chlorprothixine and thioridazine (Hollister, 1964). Most commonly agranulocytosis develops during the first 12 weeks of treatment, independent of dosage. After restarting treatment with the same agents, agranulocytosis may again flare up. These observations seem to make it likely that an immunologic reaction is responsible for the phenothiazine-induced agranulocytosis. CPZ *in vitro* inhibits the uptake of tritiated thymidine and uridine by leucocytes of patients who suffered from phenothiazine-induced agranulocytosis (Pasciotta and Kaldahl, 1962). The significance of this finding is not known.

7. Allergic Skin Reactions

While allergic skin reactions are known to occur during phenothiazine treatment, they have become rarer in recent times. Photosensitization of the skin is an interesting phenomenon for which the following explanation has been advanced by Domino (1962 b): According to Whitten and Filmer (1947), young cattle develop a keratitis after administration of phenothiazine as anthelmintic, whereas similarly treated sheep remain healthy. Moreover, it has been found that the bovine species (but not sheep!) metabolize the phenothiazine to the corresponding sulfoxide which can be detected in high concentration in the aqueous humor of the anterior eye chamber. Domino (1962 b), therefore, raises the question whether or not the individual variation in susceptibility of patients to photosensitization in response to phenothiazines could be due to differences in the metabolism of these agents.

8. Ocular Side-effects

Rare side-effects occurring during phenothiazine therapy are retinopathy with pigment deposition and iridocycloplegia. High dosage and long term treatment may lead to granular deposits in the lens and clouding of the cornea (DeLong et al., 1965).

9. Teratogenicity

Opinions differ as to whether or not ingestion of phenothiazines during pregnancy causes congenital malformations. Hollister (1964), on the basis of the available literature, concludes that there is at present no reason to assume that phenothiazine derivatives are teratogenic.

10. Danger of Suicide

Since the clinical introduction of phenothiazines, the incidence of suicide in psychiatric patients has increased sharply (Schneidman et al., 1964). However, it must be remembered that the most severe cases treated today enjoy a freedom of movement which was previously completely unknown. This may contribute to the higher suicide rate (Hollister, 1964).

11. Sudden Death

Occasionally during chronic phenothiazine treatment sudden death may occur. If this is the consequence of convulsions (see this chapter, section G, 2), the cause of death may be asphyxia due to aspiration. Hollister (1957) has reported a few cases which make it seem likely that ventricular fibrillation has to be considered as cause of sudden death. It is possible that this effect is related to the quinidine-like action of phenothiazines on the heart (compare with this chapter, section G, 8 and B, 2).

II. Butyrophenones

The butyrophenones constitute a series of potent neuroleptic compounds among which haloperidol has been the most intensively studied. The butyrophenones differ from the phenothiazine neuroleptics by the almost complete absence of effects on the peripheral autonomic nervous system. The pharmacological literature has been summarized by Janssen (1967).

A. Structure Activity Relationships

Extensive studies on the relation between structure and activity in the butyrophenone series indicate that haloperidol, although a potent neuroleptic and antiemetic of long duration, is not the most active compound in this series. Spiroperidol and droperidol, the most potent neuroleptic drugs known to date, are approximately 900 times more potent than promazine in rats and 15,000 times more potent than promazine in dogs.

B. Peripheral Effects

1. Interference with Autonomic Mediators

In contrast to reserpine and the phenothiazines, the butyrophenones have no significant influence on peripheral sympathetic or parasympathetic function. No significant effects of haloperidol on acetylcholine-induced contraction of isolated ileum, on the vasodepressor response induced by acetylcholine and on the salivation induced by pilocarpine have been found. Equally weak is the antihistamine effect of haloperidol *in vitro* and *in vivo*. The effects of norepinephrine on blood pressure and nictitating membrane of cat are not altered or only slightly depressed (Theobald et al., 1965). Alpha-adrenolytic effects are observed only after large doses of haloperidol (Janssen et al., 1965). Van Rossum (1965, 1966) demonstrated that the blood pressure fall induced in dogs by dopamine after prior blockade of α-adrenergic receptors is markedly diminished by haloperidol.

2. Cardiovascular Effects

In cats, dogs and rabbits haloperidol causes a small, though prolonged, fall in blood pressure. This is accompanied by a slight increase in heart rate and diminution of the peripheral resistance. The blood pressure fall induced by vagal nerve stimulation is not affected by haloperidol nor the blood pressure rise induced by splanchnic nerve stimulation. The carotid occlusion reflexes are diminished; the vasopressor response evoked by hypothalamic stimulation is diminished in cats and rabbits (Schmitt and Schmitt, 1962).

C. Central Effects

1. Influence at the Spinal Level

In spinal cats haloperidol inhibits the patellar reflex with a concomitant diminution of the flexor reflex. In intact cats the facilitation of the patellar reflex induced by brain stem stimulation is depressed, and the linguo-mandibular reflex is diminished. From these effects it may be concluded that haloperidol and possibly the other butyrophenones affect somatic reflexes at both the spinal and the supraspinal levels (Bhargava and Srivastava, 1965).

2. Supraspinal Effects

a) Antiemetic Effect

Behaviorally inactive parenteral or oral doses of haloperidol prevent the emetic action of apomorphine in dogs (Janssen and Niemegeers, 1959). In this respect, haloperidol is considerably more potent than chlorpromazine.

b) Interactions with Centrally Active Agents

Haloperidol antagonizes various effects of amphetamine in mice, e. g., toxicity, psychomotor stimulation and compulsory chewing (Frommel and Chmouliovsky, 1964; Theobald et al., 1965).

Tremorine-induced tremor is markedly reduced by haloperidol (Theobald et al., 1965), a finding which has not been confirmed (Spencer, 1965).

Haloperidol potentiates the hypnotic effects of ether and barbiturates but not those of morphine in mice (Boissier and Pagny, 1960). The morphine rage in cats is partially antagonized (Boissier et al., 1961).

3. Effects on Behavior

a) Effects on Innate Behavior

The butyrophenones decrease spontaneous locomotor activity and increase the tendency of rodents to maintain induced body postures (catalepsy). The CNS depressant effect of haloperidol is also demonstrated by the disruption of coordinated somatomotor activity in the rotarod test (Janssen, 1961). Mice rendered aggressive by isolation exhibit reduced fighting behavior after administration of butyrophenones (Janssen, 1960).

b) Effects on Operant Behavior

Squirrel monkeys on a Sidman avoidance schedule exhibit marked anti-avoidance activity after administration of neuroleptic agents, haloperidol being approximately 7 times more potent than chlorpromazine (Hanson et al., 1966). Like other neuroleptics, haloperidol also increases active avoidance failures in rats, whereas the ability to refrain from an action inducing punishment (passive avoidance) is not significantly altered (Morpurgo, 1965). Similarly, haloperidol inhibits conditioned shock avoidance behavior in the "jumping box" test (Niemegeers and Janssen, 1965). Self-stimulation of the medial forebrain bundle in rats is greatly reduced by small doses of butyrophenones, haloperidol being more active than chlorpromazine (Dresse, 1966).

D. Biochemical Effects

1. Interaction with Adrenergic Mediators

Like other neuroleptic agents, butyrophenones also interfere with central adrenergic mechanisms. Thus haloperidol, among other butyrophenones, counteracts the increase in rat brain NE induced by MAO-inhibitors (Dresse, 1966), whereas the depleting effect of reserpine is not influenced (Dresse and DeMeyer, 1964). Small doses of haloperidol also enhance the accumulation of o-methylated norepinephrine metabolites brought about by monoamine-oxidase inhibition (Carlsson and Lindqvist, 1963). Like phenothiazines, butyrophenones interfere with dopamine metabolism, increasing the concentration of homovanillic acid in the caudate nucleus (Andén et al., 1964 b; Sharman, 1966). Haloperidol antagonizes the vasodepressor effect of dopamine (Van Rossum, 1966). This dopamine blockade may be of importance in the mechanism of the central action of haloperidol, particularly on the extrapyramidal centers (Van Rossum, 1967). In this respect, it is of note that in dogs, the dopamine content of the caudate nucleus is significantly diminished by haloperidol (Himwich and Glisson, 1967).

2. Metabolic Fate

The excretion pattern and metabolic pathway of haloperidol in rats and dogs are similar. Randomly labelled, tritiated haloperidol administered by the parenteral route or gavage is rapidly absorbed in 24 hours. The highest amount of radioactivity is found in the liver, whereas only 0.1% (out of a total recovery of 82%) is present in brain. The major metabolic pathway is by oxidative N-dealkylation yielding β-(p-fluorobenzoyl)-propionic acid and p-fluorophenacetinic acid (Soudijn et al., 1967; Braun and Poos, 1966). The above metabolites are devoid of neuroleptic activity in rodents and dogs.

E. Adverse Reactions and Dangers

1. Extrapyramidal Side-effects. Most frequently observed during haloperidol treatment are extrapyramidal signs of parkinson-like type, including akathisia, dystonia and tremor. These symptoms are dose-related and can be reversed by lowering dosage or temporarily discontinuing therapy.

2. Other Central Side-effects. Confusion, convulsions and stupor have been reported but seem to occur rarely.

3. Autonomic Side-effects. Hypotension, tachycardia, gastrointestinal disturbances and vomiting as well as dryness of oral mucosa have been noted but are relatively infrequent.

4. Other Side-effects. Rare cases of leukopenia have been described. Liver impairment with and without jaundice has been noted, the overall incidence being approximately 2 per thousand patients.

III. Reserpine and Reserpine-like Agents

In spite of the fact that the principal alkaloid of the Indian plant, Rauwolfia serpentina (Benth), has only recently been described by Müller, Schlittler and Bein (1952), the literature is already so extensive that it is impossible to present an exhaustive account. During the past ten years numerous reviews in English, German and French have appeared. Bein (1956) and Werner (1954) mention reports on the first experiments by Siddiqui and Siddiqui in which an attempt was made to isolate active components from the plant used as a calming drug in Indian folk medicine. They also refer to the first Indian pharmacological investigations of Chopra, Gupta and Raymond-Hamet who described the hypotensive effect of Rauwolfia. Woodson et al. (1957) report on the botany and pharmacognosy of the plant.

In 1955 several groups of investigators disclosed the chemical structure (Huebner et al., 1955; Huebner and Wenkert, 1955; Diassi et al., 1955; Van Tamelen and Hance, 1955). Woodward et al. (1958) completed the total synthesis.

A. Structure-activity Relationships

There are numerous naturally occurring and semisynthetic reserpine derivatives with pharmacological and biochemical actions similar to the parent substance. Furthermore, there are synthetic analogs belonging to the group of benzoquinolizines which also possess reserpine-like activity.

Removal of the 3,4,5-trimethoxybenzoyl rest and demethylation leads to reserpic acid which is, like methyl reserpate, inactive. The introduction of acid groups, other than trimethoxybenzoic acid, also diminishes its effectiveness. Minor substitutions on the trimethoxybenzoic acid moiety lead to agents such as rescinnamine and syrosingopine in which activity is retained but is weaker than in reserpine. Within a restricted dose range syrosingopine is more effective peripherally than centrally (Orlans et al., 1960). Neither the 11-methoxy nor the 17-methyl group is necessary for reserpine-like activity. Thus, the naturally occurring alkaloid raunescine and the semi-synthetic derivative, 11-desmethoxy-reserpine (deserpidine), are pharmacologically and biochemically reserpine-like in their effects. However, isoraunescine is inactive. Methoserpidine, in which the methoxy-group is in the 10 position instead of the 11 position, is an active analog although its effects appear to be predominantly peripheral in some species (Gros et al., 1959; Sanan and Vogt, 1962).

The series of synthetic reserpine analogs, all having the benzoquinolizine structure, is of interest. Among these compounds tetrabenazine is best known. Tetrabenazine possesses reserpine-like activity which is, in contrast to reserpine, of short duration (Pletscher et al., 1958; Quinn et al., 1959). Theoretically interesting are the two derivatives RO 4-1284 and RO 4-1398. According to Pletscher et al. (1959 b), the former is more effective as a tranquilizer and releaser of brain NE than RO 4-1398, whereas both compounds reduce cerebral 5-HT to the same extent. These results were disputed by Brodie et al. (1960). For theoretical significance of these findings, see this chapter, section C, 1 a, β.

Most frequently used clinically are reserpine, deserpidine, rescinnamine and syrosingopine.

B. Peripheral Effects

1. Influence on the Peripheral Sympathetic Nervous System

Reserpine and most reserpine-like agents release norepinephrine, the transmitter substance of postganglionic sympathetic nerves, from all parts of the postsynaptic nervous tissue (ganglion cells, nerve fibers, nerve terminals). Consequently, after injection of several doses of reserpine, the neuron is depleted of its transmitter substance. If the norepinephrine depletion is extensive, transmission of postganglionic impulses to the effector organ is no longer possible, whereas the transmission from pre- to postganglionic neurons remains intact. Therefore, the response of the effector organ to pre-, or postganglionic electrical stimulation is abolished (Muscholl and Vogt, 1957 a; Carlsson et al., 1957 b; Burn and Rand, 1958; Trendelenburg und Gravenstein, 1958). This effect is only achieved if the norepinephrine depletion exceeds 70% to 80%. It should be also noted that NE-depletion of sympathetically innervated structures is not the only preequisite for reserpine to be effective at the end-organ. Thus, the norepinephrine content of sympathetic ganglion cells reaches a minimum 3—4 hours after reserpine administration, but the blockade of transmission is not fully developed until 24 hours later (Muscholl and Vogt, 1958). Although the significance of this time factor is not quite clear, it must be assumed that in spite of the diminution of the overall NE content, sufficient NE is present in the nerve terminals to maintain transmission shortly after reserpine injection.

Muscholl and Vogt (1958) found that reserpine releases NE from postganglionic fibers even when they are disconnected from the preganglionic fibers. These authors therefore postulate that the reserpine action is purely peripheral. However, the reserpine-effect seems to be prevented by ganglionic blocking agents (Kärki et al., 1959; Hertting et al., 1962), and recently Fischer et al. (1965 b) reported on a similar, though very weak, effect after cutting preganglionic fibers.

The diminished activity of the postganglionic adrenergic neuron after reserpine administration is accompanied by a hypersensitivity of adrenergically innervated structures to direct-acting sympathomimetics such as epinephrine, norepinephrine, dopamine, epinine and others (see Bein et al., 1953). This phenomenon resembles denervation hypersensitivity in adrenergically innervated organs. The common denominator of both effects is the depletion of the transmitter substance in peripheral nervous structures (NE) by reserpine and by degeneration of norepinephrine containing nerve fibers following denervation.

The term "stores" or "storage sites" coined by Burn (1960) is important for the understanding of the mechanism of hypersensitivity. It refers to the ability of adrenergic nerve terminals to take up exogenous or endogenously-released norepinephrine and to store it. According to Burn (1960) and other authors, this is one of the more important mechanisms by which norepinephrine is inactivated. Elimination of the storage sites, either by degeneration of the postganglionic neuron or by inhibiting storage *per se* with reserpine (see this chapter, section B, 4 b), leads to a flooding of the receptors when norepinephrine is administered and consequently to an increased response ("hypersensitivity") of these receptors to the exogenous norepinephrine. In this connection therefore, "hypersensitivity" means "diminished biological inactivation" resulting in increased effectiveness. However, Trendelenburg (1963), in a critical review of the problem of decreased and increased sensitivity of sympathetically innervated structures, has cited data which do not permit unconditional acceptance of the simple hypothesis advanced above. It is, therefore, advisable to leave open the possibility that denervation of adrenergic receptors causes hypersensitivity similar to that seen after denervation of striated muscle in response to acetylcholine.

Muscholl (1960) has shown that the uptake of circulating norepinephrine into sympathetically innervated organs (e. g., rat heart *in vivo*) is markedly reduced by reserpine. This important observation has subsequently been confirmed many times (Hertting et al., 1961; Crout et al., 1962; Andén et al., 1963 a; Inouye and Tanaka, 1964). It is also probable that endogenously formed catecholamines cannot be retained in the storage sites after reserpine treatment. Andén et al. (1964 a) believe that this reserpine-induced inhibition of storage ability of peripheral adrenergic neurons reflects their functional blockade much better than the degree of norepinephrine depletion itself. The possibility that the catecholamine releasing effect of reserpine is due to inhibition of storage ability is discussed in this section part 4 b.

2. Catecholamine Release from the Adrenal Medulla

Holzbauer and Vogt (1956), and Carlsson and Hillarp (1956) were the first to observe that reserpine depletes norepinephrine in the adrenal medulla of cats and rabbits. This observation has subsequently been confirmed for all species examined. However, the sensitivity of various species differs greatly and decreases in the following order: rabbit > cat > rat > chicken. Two mechanisms seem to play a role in the liberation of catecholamines from the adrenal medulla: a central mechanism with catecholamines released by stimulation of the splanchnic nerves, and a peripheral mechanism with the direct action of reserpine on the chromaffin cells of the medulla. The central mechanism is far more sensitive in that only very small doses of reserpine are required to elicit it in rabbits (Kroneberg and Schümann, 1957, 1958), whereas considerably larger doses are necessary to induce the direct release of amines. However, species differences determine the extent of the neuronally elicited catecholamine depletion. In cats, the depletion induced by 2.5 mg/kg of reserpine is prevented by cutting the splanchnic nerves (Holzbauer and Vogt, 1956). In rabbits, sectioning the splanchnic nerves has no effect (Carlsson and Hillarp, 1956), whereas no depletion takes place when the spinal cord is transected at C_6 (Kroneberg and Schümann, 1957) or Th_1 (Takemoto et al., 1957). Denervation of the adrenal medulla of rats has no influence on reserpine-induced catecholamine depletion (Kroneberg and Schümann, 1957). These seemingly contradictory results may be explained by the assumption that in most species, after giving large doses of reserpine (more than 5 mg/kg), the peripheral mechanism plays the major role in catecholamine depletion (cf. Callingham and Mann, 1962).

The peripheral effect of reserpine is not due to direct inhibition of synthesis or activation of metabolizing enzymes. According to Kirshner (1962 a, b) reserpine inhibits the ability of the granules of chromaffin cells to take up and bind catecholamines against a concentration gradient ("inhibition of storage capability"). (See also this part, section 4, b.)

If the alkaloid is repeatedly administered in small, daily doses, the catecholamine depletion of the adrenal medulla is more pronounced than after injection of one large dose (Muscholl and Vogt, 1958). After administration of a single dose of reserpine, the depletion, which reaches a maximum after 16 hours (Callingham and Mann, 1962), is of unusually long duration. In rabbits the normal catecholamine content is reached one to two weeks after injection (Muscholl and Vogt, 1958), and in chickens several months (!) are required for full recovery (Burack et al., 1960).

There is no unanimous opinion in the literature regarding the question as to whether or not both epinephrine and norepinephrine are liberated by reserpine to the same extent. Stjärne and Shapiro (1958), and Cammanni et al. (1958) report that norepinephrine is released preferentially, whereas Coupland (1958), Mirkin (1958) and Callingham and Mann (1962) find no actual proof for this supposition.

It is noteworthy that after reserpine-induced depletion, the resynthesis of norepinephrine and epinephrine takes place at different rates. There is a shift in favor of norepinephrine after chronic administration of reserpine (Muscholl and Vogt, 1958) and during the re-covery phase (Callingham and Mann, 1962). This demonstrates that the resynthesis of norepinephrine occurs relatively rapidly, whereas its methylation to epinephrine is a much slower process.

Bertler et al. (1961) have accumulated data which make it likely that, similar to the adrenergic neuron, the uptake of newly formed dopamine and norepinephrine into the granules of the chromaffin cells of the adrenal medulla is prevented after reserpine administration. In rabbits, DOPA administration usually leads to a marked uptake of newly synthesized norepinephrine and dopamine into the granules. This does not occur in reserpine-pretreated animals. For these reasons, it is assumed that the catecholamine-releasing effect of reserpine is generally due to an inhibition of catecholamine uptake into storage sites (see this section, part 4 b).

3. Reserpine-induced Release of 5-Hydroxytryptamine

Reserpine releases 5-HT from all tissues containing it. This process is particularly pronounced in blood platelets and the gastrointestinal tract.

a) Blood Platelets

5-HT is released *in vitro* and *in vivo* by very small doses of reserpine. In rabbits i. v. injection of 0.015 mg/kg reduced 5-HT in blood by 75% (Shore et al., 1956 a; Naess and Schanche, 1956). In man, a similar dose (1 mg total ∼0.015 mg/kg i. m.) causes an almost complete disappearance of 5-HT from blood platelets (Hardisty et al., 1956). The sensitivity of other species (guinea pigs, rats, pigeons) is about 10 times less. Maximal depletion of blood platelets is generally reached 16 hours after reserpine injection. After 2—3 days recovery sets in and, depending on the species, normal 5-HT concen-trations are re-established 1—3 weeks later.

Reserpine does not only release 5-HT from blood platelets but also prevents its uptake. If blood platelets of man or rabbit are pretreated for 1 to 9 days and then suspended in a 5-HT-containing medium, they take up 75—90% less 5-HT than platelets from untreated con-trols (Hardisty et al., 1956; Brodie et al., 1957).

The release of 5-HT from blood platelets is not simply a process of displacement. It is known from *in vitro* experiments that one molecule of reserpine can release hundreds of 5-HT molecules (Shore et al., 1956 b). *In vitro*, concentrations of as little as $0.05 \gamma/ml$ of reserpine are effective and a maximal depletion is achieved with only 0.3 γ/ml.

b) Gastrointestinal Tract

Pletscher et al. (1955) first observed that reserpine releases 5-HT from the enterochromaffin cells of rabbits. This finding has since been repeatedly confirmed. The sensitivity of the gastrointestinal tract is, however, considerably less than that of blood platelets. Therefore, it is possible to deplete blood platelets of 5-HT with small doses of reserpine without affecting the gastrointestinal 5-HT content (Waalkes et al., 1957).

Zbinden et al. (1957 a) noted considerable regional differences of sensitivity towards reserpine in rabbits. Thus the fundus of the stomach is resistant to reserpine whereas the mucosa of the pre-pyloric area and the ileum are equally sensitive. Again, species differences exist in that rabbits, guinea pigs and chickens are far more sensitive than rats, which only respond with a moderate depletion of gastrointestinal 5-HT in spite of large doses of reserpine.

In vitro, even large doses of reserpine do not release 5-HT from the isolated guinea pig ileum (Benditt, 1957).

4. Mechanism of the Amine-liberating Effect of Reserpine

a) General Comments

A considerable portion of norepinephrine and epinephrine of the adrenal medulla, the adrenergic nerves and sympathetically innervated organs is contained in specific storage granules (Blaschko and Welch, 1953; Hillarp et al., 1953; von Euler and Hillarp, 1956; Schümann, 1958 a). 5-HT of blood platelets (Baker et al., 1959) and enterochromaffin cells also appears to be concentrated in granules (Baker, 1958; Prusoff, 1960). The granules are organelles which are morphologically and biochemically different from mitochondria. The granules of adrenergic nerves and sympathetically innervated organs measure 300—2000 Å; those of the adrenal medulla, 500—6000 Å.

On the basis of the finding that the specific catecholamine (and also probably 5-HT) granules contain large amounts of adenosine triphosphate (ATP), it has been concluded (Blaschko et al., 1956; see for further literature Hagen and Barnett, 1960) that the catecholamines, being present in the granules in a strongly hypertonic concentration, are retained and stored in iso-osmotic condition by binding to ATP. In favor of this binding mechanism is the finding that the molar ratio of catecholamines to ATP in the granules of adrenal medulla is 4 : 1, four being the number of free valences of ATP available for binding of catecholamines. Philippu and Schümann (1963) have recently considered the possibility that the ATP present in catecholamine granules is somehow anchored to the ribonucleic acid of the granules.

It is important to recall that the granules are not only the substrate for storing catecholamines but also the place of synthesis. According to Kirshner (1957) and Blaschko (1959), norepinephrine is not formed in the cell plasma but originates from dopamine within the granules. Dopamine itself, however, is formed in the cell plasma from L-DOPA by decarboxylation.

The catecholamine content in granules varies depending on the tissue. In the adrenal medulla it is 70—80% of the total catecholamine concentration (Blaschko and Welch, 1953; Hillarp et al., 1953; Hillarp, 1960 b), in the extraterminal portions of adrenergic nerves approximately 30% and in sympathetically innervated organs up to 70%. The fact that catecholamines exist in a bound and free state within the same cell makes it likely that two functionally different "pools" will be revealed by drugs acting on the adrenergic neuron and by nerve stimulation. It must be assumed that there is an equilibrium between the two amine storage sites in that amines released from extragranular sites are constantly replaced by intragranular amines, and the intragranular amines are then replaced by resynthesis.

Important for the understanding of the processes taking place at the adrenergic nerve ending is the fact that the nerve ending not only releases the transmitter but also reabsorbs it. This reuptake guarantees the "economic use" of amines. Paton (1960) was the first to postulate clearly such a function for the adrenergic nerve ending; this concept is related to that of the "storage sites", a term coined by Burn (1960). Hertting and Axelrod (1961) and later Hukovic and Muscholl (1962) have adduced experimental evidence for this hypothesis.

b) Effect of Reserpine

In general, it is possible to distinguish three fundamentally different processes involved in the release of amines from storage sites: 1. active release from granules; 2. blockade of amine uptake into granules; 3. blockade of reuptake of released amines from the extraneuronal environment.

The latter two mechanisms appear to be most important for the reserpine-induced amine depletion. Most investigators assume that blockade of amine uptake into the granules is the key process.

This viewpoint is supported by considerable evidence:

1. It is almost certain that reserpine does not induce an active amine release from granules. To effect release from isolated granules *in vitro*, extremely high doses of reserpine are required, concentrations which are hardly attained *in vivo*. This has been repeatedly demonstrated using granules isolated from various organs (for literature see Stjärne, 1964).

2. On the other hand, very low concentrations of reserpine inhibit the uptake of catecholamines into granules isolated from the adrenal medulla (Kirshner, 1962 a, b; Carlsson et al., 1962) and adrenergic nerves (von Euler and Lishajko, 1963). The same effect has been observed in granules derived from animals which were pretreated with reserpine (Kirshner et al., 1963). Furthermore, the previously mentioned experiments of Bertler et al. (1961) show that reserpine inhibits the uptake of catecholamines formed from L-DOPA into the granules of the adrenal medulla.

Inhibition of amine uptake into granules has two consequences: a) After reserpine treatment, the amines are more vulnerable to enzymatic destruction by MAO; b) the synthesis of NE from dopamine, taking place within the granules (vide this section, a), is inhibited. It seems that this inhibition of norepinephrine formation in the granules is responsible for reserpine-induced depletion of NE stores since the physiologically released NE cannot be replaced (Kirshner, 1962 a, b).

3. Stjärne believes that, in addition to the above described mechanisms, a blockade of the axonal membrane for catecholamines is important for reserpine-induced depletion of many tissues (e. g., heart). This viewpoint is supported by Stjärne's (1964) own data and the findings of other investigators who have shown that reserpine inhibits uptake of amines into blood platelets (Hughes and Brodie, 1959), heart and brain tissues (Campos and Shideman, 1962; Dengler et al., 1962) as a result of blockade of cell membrane permeability. According to Stjärne (1964), it is possible that in organs with high sympathetic activity reuptake of physiologically released transmitter is an important mechanism for maintaining the intraneuronal norepinephrine concentration. The inhibition of this mechanism by reserpine consequently would lead to an exhaustion of the norepinephrine stores.

Recent pharmacological experiments by Lindmar and Muscholl (1964), Carlsson and Waldeck (1965), and histochemical studies by

Malmfors (1965) (see also further literature) make it highly probable that *inhibition of uptake into granules and storage* of catecholamines represents the principal mechanism of the depleting action of reserpine.

Simultaneously with the release of intragranular amines, ATP also disappears from the granules. Thus, the molar ratio between amines and ATP generally remains the same (Schümann, 1958 b; Kirpekar et al., 1958; Hillarp, 1960 a). However, some findings indicate that reserpine treatment may shift the ratio in favor of ATP in that the release of amines is greater than that of ATP (Burack et al., 1960) or that ATP is more rapidly resynthesized than catecholamines (Schümann, 1958 b).

5. Peripheral Consequences of the Biochemical Effects of Reserpine

Almost all reserpine effects, with the exception of those affecting the CNS, can be explained as hypofunction of the sympathetic nervous system, e. g., miosis, ptosis, enophthalmus, bradycardia and hypotension. Reserpine is devoid of ganglionic blocking effect. If the norepinephrine stores are completely depleted, the response to preganglionic and postganglionic stimulation of adrenergic nerves is obliterated. As early as 1955, Bein reported that reserpine blocks the carotid sinus pressor response without affecting the afferent (baro-receptors) portion of this reflex. Vagally induced respiratory reflexes are not altered by reserpine. McQueen (1956) found that the vasodilating effect of reserpine is abolished after sympathectomy. However, one has to keep in mind that the influence of reserpine on sympathetic centers in the hypothalamus appears first, and only later followed, particularly during prolonged treatment, by the peripheral effects.

The depletion of catecholamine stores is a slow process, and most of the amines are destroyed by MAO before they can exert an effect. Nevertheless, Plummer et al. (1954) observed tachycardia in the heart-lung preparation of the dog shortly after reserpine injection. In the same preparation, Krayer (1958) and coworkers (Innes et al., 1958; Krayer and Fuentes (1958); Paasonen and Krayer (1958)) found that reserpine and other rauwolfia alkaloids (raunescine, deserpidine and rescinnamine) first cause tachycardia and shortening of conduction time, later followed by bradycardia and a prolongation of conduction time. The two latter effects only occur at the commencement of treatment with those alkaloids which posses antifibrillatory activity such as ajmaline, serpentine, aricine, reserpinine and yohimbine. Initial vasopressor responses to reserpine are often noted (De Jongh and Van Proosdij-Hartzema, 1955; Maxwell et al., 1957; Domino and Rech, 1957). If experimental animals are spinalized or pretreated with cocaine, signs of sympathetic stimulation become particularly evident after reserpine injection, the effect being due to a release of catecholamines (Schneider and Rinehart, 1956; Horita, 1958). The vasopressor effect of reserpine, which occurs after pretreatment with MAO-inhibitors, is based on the same mechanism of action (Chessin et al., 1957).

In agreement with these pharmacological results are the findings of Muscholl and Vogt (1957 b) who observed an increase in plasma epinephrine concentration in rabbits 100 minutes after reserpine administration. In contrast, the catecholamine level decreases after chronic treatment in man (Burger, 1957). An initial increase of urinary catecholamines is also observed (Birke et al., 1957), generally followed by a decrease of epinephrine and norepinephrine excretion (Gaddum et al., 1958; Kuschke and von Ditfurth, 1958). However, Carlsson et al. (1959 b) have only noted a decrease in norepinephrine excretion.

It has been stated already that the catecholamines released by reserpine are increasingly exposed to enzymatic destruction by MAO. Therefore an increase in desaminated metabolites is found in heart and urine (Kopin et al., 1962; Nash et al., 1963; Kopin and Gordon, 1962, 1963).

After a varying latency following reserpine injection, the effects of epinephrine, NE and isoproterenol are enhanced. The time for the development of maximal hypersensitivity of the nictitating membrane is approximately 14 days (Fleming and Trendelenburg, 1961) and of the heart, 2—3 days (Bejrablaya et al., 1958), whereas development of maximal blood pressure responses is reached much earlier (Burn and Rand, 1958). The potentiation of catecholamine effects in acute experiments is probably not due to hypersensitivity but represents in all likelihood an additive effect of the reserpine-released and injected catecholamines (Trendelenburg, 1963). Organs rendered hypersensitive to catecholamines by reserpine respond like denervated tissues which are also devoid of amines (von Euler and Purkhold, 1951; Goodall, 1951; Burn and Rand, 1959). However, a strict parallelism between reserpine-induced depletion of catecholamine stores and hypersensitivity cannot be established. The depletion appears to precede the development of hypersensitivity. However, there is undoubtedly a connection between the two processes. Moore and Moran (1962) have found that only the chronotropic effect of norepinephrine on the heart is enhanced but not the inotropic effect (compare also Trendelenburg and Gravenstein, 1958). It is certain that reserpine is not an adrenolytic agent. It neither affects the enzymes responsible for the catecholamine synthesis (compare, however, this section, part 4 b, 2) nor the effect of the chemical transmitter.

From the above mentioned findings, it is not surprising that reserpine causes a dominance of the parasympathetic system. Brücke and Spring (1963) observed that sphincter spasm develops in the rabbit cardia within a few minutes after i. v. injection of reserpine similar to the spasms occurring after ganglionic blockers or denervation of adrenergic fibers. Atropine blocks this spasm. An increase in bladder tonus (Maxwell et al., 1956) and micturition difficulties after reserpine administration may be similarly explained. It is not necessary to postulate a direct stimulating effect of reserpine-released 5-TH on central parasympathetic mechanisms (Brodie et al., 1959 a). The vasodepressor effect of reserpine is not blocked by atropine (Bein et al., 1953).

Another effect of reserpine-released catecholamines (and perhaps some metabolic products with more pronounced β-type activity) is the often observed initial hyperglycemia which was first described by Kuschke and Frantz (1955).

Other pharmacological results can also be easily explained by reserpine-induced depletion of NE and perhaps also of 5-HT stores. Thus, Burn and Rand (1958) have demonstrated in spinal cats that tyramine, phenylethylamine, phenylethanolamine, amphetamine and ephedrine fail to raise the blood pressure after reserpine-pretreatment. Furthermore, these indirectly acting sympathomimetic agents also fail to evoke contractions of the nictitating membrane and spleen in reserpine-treated animals. In isolated atria, Holtz et al. (1960) and Kuschinsky et al. (1960) have found that tyramine is devoid of positiv chronotropic and inotropic activity after reserpine-pretreatment. Similar results have been obtained by Gaffney (1962) *in vivo* (compare also Trendelenburg, 1961) and by Bejrablaya et al. (1958) in the dog heart-lung preparation. The ineffectiveness of indirectly acting sympathomimetics under these conditions is due to the fact that these agents do not directly react with adrenergic receptors but release amines (epinephrine, NE and perhaps dopamine) from the stores, though by a mechanism different from that of reserpine. After complete depletion, these agents are deprived of their mediator. Burn and Rand

(1958) documented this assumption in showing that the sensitivity to tyramine in reserpine-treated animals can be restored by infusions of NE. Similar results have been reported by Kuschinsky et al. (1960) in regard to the isolated heart muscle preparation. Lindmar and Muscholl (1961) demonstrated that neither tyramine nor 1-dimethyl-4-phenylpiperazine release NE from the heart after reserpine-pretreatment. Schümann and Philippu (1961) have presented direct evidence for the NE-releasing effect of tyramine by showing that this amine releases NE from isolated granules by stoichiometric displacement (for further references see Stjärne, 1964).

As early as 1956, in the review of Bein, the effects of reserpine on the gastrointestinal tract are extensively discussed. Recently, Emås (1963) has reinvestigated the influence of reserpine on gastric secretion in cats and found that histamine- and gastrin-induced secretion are enhanced, whereas methacholine- or insulin-elicited secretion are diminished. In man, a daily dose of 0.75 to 1.0 mg of reserpine has a secretagogue effect on the stomach. Large doses may even be ulcerogenic. It appears impossible to decide whether or not the hypersecretory and ulcerogenic effect is causally related to release of 5-HT. 5-HT and 5-HTP can produce gastric ulcers in rats (Haverback and Bogdanski, 1957), but, in contrast to reserpine, these two agents inhibit gastric secretion (Haverback and Wirtschafter, 1962). On the other hand, increased intestinal mobility and diarrhea after reserpine administration is possibly due to locally accumulated 5-HT (Bein, 1956). This is particularly likely since similar symptoms occur in cases of carcinoid tumors which contain large amounts of 5-HT (Lembeck, 1953).

It appears that the ulcerogenic and secretagogue effect of reserpine may be better related to its histamine-releasing properties (Haverback and Wirtschafter, 1962). The results of Kim and Shore (1963) corroborate this view. Histamine is also liberated by reserpine from mast cells of rabbits and guinea pigs (Waalkes and Weissbach, 1956; Waalkes et al., 1959) but not of rats (Bhattacharya and Lewis, 1956; Moran and Westerholm, 1963).

Also of interest is the presence and function of catecholamines in the interscapular gland (brown fat), especially in hibernating animals. In this tissue, reserpine also causes amine release and thus influences fat mobilization (Paoletti and Vertua, 1964; Stock and Westermann, 1963).

C. Central Effects
1. Biochemical Effects in CNS

Since reserpine also has several marked biochemical effects on the CNS, it appears appropriate to first discuss this aspect of central reserpine action.

a) Influence on Norepinephrine, Dopamine and 5-HT Metabolism in Brain

In analogy to the peripheral effects, the most conspicuous biochemical effect of reserpine and reserpine-like agents in the CNS is the release of NE, dopamine and 5-HT from the brain. After prolonged and intensive treatment with reserpine, the brain is depleted of these amines. Many investigators attempted to explain the central effects of this alkaloid with this principal biochemical action. All such attempts presume that these amines play a physiological role, probably as transmitter substances, in the functioning of certain CNS systems. In the experimental and theoretical literature, three principal hypotheses stand out: α) the 5-HT-hypothesis; β) the NE-hypothesis and γ) the dopamine-hypothesis. In the following paragraphs, these three hypotheses are briefly presented to facilitate the understanding of the reserpine literature.

α) The 5-HT-hypothesis. The original hypothesis of the physiological significance of 5-HT in the CNS was based on the following observations: 1. 5-HT is present in brain tissue of all vertebrates in a characteristic regional distribution pattern. The highest concentration is found in the limbic system (Twarog and Page, 1953; Amin et al., 1954; Paasonen and Vogt, 1956; Bogdanski et al., 1957) an area involved in the regulation of emotional behavior. 2. Lysergic acid diethylamide (LSD), which causes marked psychic changes in man (LSD-psychoses), is a strong peripheral 5-HT antagonist (Gaddum and Hameed, 1954). Therefore, it has been assumed (but not proven) that the central actions of LSD are also due to its 5-HT antagonistic properties and, consequently, that cerebral 5-HT must play a role in psychological processes (Gaddum, 1957; Woolley and Shaw, 1954, 1957). Such an assumption is untenable in view of the fact that other LSD-analogues which also are 5-HT antagonists (e. g., Brom-LSD) do not induce mental disturbances. Furthermore, this hypothesis is difficult to reconcile with the finding that in high doses, 5-HTP, the precursor of 5-HT, induces a central stimulation resembling that elicited by LSD (Bogdanski et al., 1958).

Since reserpine liberates 5-HT from brain (Pletscher et al., 1956; Paasonen and Vogt, 1956), Brodie and coworkers postulated that the reserpine-induced sedation is due to continuous release of small but pharmacologically active quantities of 5-HT. Arguments in favor of this view have been reviewed by Brodie et al. (1959 a), Brodie and Costa (1962) and Brodie et al. (1960). From numerous ingenious experiments, presenting however mostly indirect evidence, Brodie concluded that 5-HT is the modulator, if not the transmitter substance, of the "endophylactic trophotropic" system of W. R. Hess. This would explain the central and peripheral parasympathetic predominance after reserpine treatment. The finding that in many species after pretreatment with MAO-inhibitors reserpine causes stimulation instead of sedation (see chapter IV, section C, 1 e and 2 a, E) cannot be readily reconciled with Brodie's viewpoints. Brodie speculates that by inhibiting the metabolism of 5-HT with MAO-inhibitors reserpine releases quantities of cerebral 5-HT so large that a paradoxical stimulation of central synapses occurs. At present, Brodie's conclusions should be regarded as hypothetical. An increasing amount of data indicates that reserpine sedation may be linked to catecholamine depletion in certain brain regions (Carlsson, 1961; Matsuoka et al., 1964). However, Matussek and Patschke (1964) have recently made an observation which does not contradict Brodie's hypothesis. These authors have found that in golden hamsters the concentration of brain 5-HT increases during sleep, whereas the NE content is slightly decreased. During wakefulness and slight activity both amines are in equilibrium, whereas marked motor hyperactivity produces a fall in 5-HT content.

Wooley and Shaw (1957) have suggested that cerebral 5-HT influences the mobility of oligodendroglia. In tissue cultures glial cells constantly exhibit pulsating movements which in the brain, may be important for the distribution of metabolic products in the extracellular compartments. It has been observed that 5-HT causes contractions of the oligodendroglia cells, thus increasing their pulsations. This effect could, according to Woolley, cause changes in cerebral metabolism and consequently alter brain function.

β) *The Norepinephrine-hypothesis.* Many publications deal with the question of the physiological significance of NE in brain. The fact that NE is particularly concentrated in the central areas representing the sympathetic system (hypothalamus, central grey of mesencephalon, floor of fourth ventricle, reticular formation) suggests that

NE is important for the functioning of these areas (Vogt, 1954). This assumption is corroborated by the finding that agents (insulin, nicotine, morphine, β-tetrahydronaphthylamine, picrotoxin, apomorphine and ether) which stimulate central adrenergic mechanisms release NE from the hypothalamus with a consequent diminution by 50% of NE content in this area (Vogt, 1954, 1957). Moreover, MAO-inhibitors which cause an increase in brain NE-content also have central stimulant effects (vide chapter V, section C, 2 a). It can be assumed that the NE which is continuously released is protected from breakdown by the MAO-inhibitors and therefore accumulates and becomes more effective.

Large doses of reserpine cause an almost complete depletion of brain NE (Holzbauer and Vogt, 1956) concomitant with marked sedation which appears to be the opposite of central sympathetic stimulation. Therefore, a significant reduction of NE concentration in the sympathetic centers leads to a cessation of their activity. Consequently, there appears to be a close relationship between the activity of the central representation of the sympathetic system, the cerebral state of excitation and the NE content of the corresponding brain regions. This viewpoint is based on the assumption that most, if not all, NE is contained in these sympathetic "centers". However, in spite of the attractive simplicity of this hypothesis, it is difficult to accept it unconditionally for the following reasons: Small doses of reserpine, which diminish the NE content in the hypothalamus to the same extent as a certain dose of picrotoxin or β-tetrahydronaphthyl-amine (Vogt, 1957), always cause sedation, whereas the latter two agents always exert a stimulant effect. In addition, after chronic reserpine treatment, causing almost complete depletion of NE, the sympathetic "centers" are functioning normally as judged by the unaltered electrical activity of the preganglionic sympathetic nerves (Iggo and Vogt, 1960). These findings indicate that the central depressant effect of reserpine is not necessarily associated with hypo-function of sympathetic centers. Therefore, the role of NE in the functioning of these centers remains hypothetical. Furthermore, the noradrenergic nature of sympathetic centers has not been unequivocally established.

It would, however, be incorrect to conclude from the described results that no relationship exists between reserpine sedation and NE-content in brain. It appears that the central representations of peripheral sympathetic mechanisms must be distinguished from the arousal mechanisms in brain. Thus, recent histochemical investigations show that NE is localized in the hypothalamus and brain stem at synapses which belong to functionally different systems; this means that the cellular distribution of NE is not restricted to areas representing sympathetic centers (Carlsson, 1964). Therefore, it is not permissible to draw conclusions from the presence of NE in the hypothalamus or reticular formation in regard to the function of a single system, unless the NE content were investigated separately in the functionally different systems of this area.

There are several pharmacological findings which do, in fact, point to a relationship between brain arousal mechanisms and NE: 1. Intravenous injection of sympathomimetic agents such as NE, amphetamine, ephedrine and L-DOPA evokes an EEG "arousal reaction" (vide Rothballer, 1959). 2. Amphetamine and L-DOPA antagonize reserpine-sedation (Tripod et al., 1954; Carlsson et al., 1957; Blaschko and Chrusciel, 1960). 3. L-DOPA increases cerebral NE-content, particularly after pretreatment with MAO-inhibitors (see Carlsson, 1959). 4. Of two benzoquinolizine derivatives with reserpine-like action only the compound with a sedative effect lowers cerebral NE, whereas 5-HT is diminished to the same extent by both drugs (Pletscher et al., 1959 b; compare with Brodie et al., 1960). Of importance is the observation of Spector et al. (1965) that the tyrosine hydroxylase inhibitor, α-methyl-p-tyrosine, which selectively depletes NE and dopamine but not 5-HT from brain, causes sedation when given chronically. The latter observation makes it unlikely that 5-HT is involved in this central depressant effect. It also indicates that in contrast to Brodie's hypothesis, the continuous release of small quantities of cerebral amines cannot be responsible for the sedative effect of reserpine, since treatment with α-methyl-p-tyrosine does not induce active release of NE or dopamine but depletes these amines as a consequence of the inhibition of their synthesis.

Data obtained by altering the NE concentration in brain with agents such as L-DOPA, MAO-inhibitors, reserpine or α-methyl-p-tyrosine have to be interpreted with caution since these agents may also influence the metabolism of dopamine or 5-HT. Thus, based on experiments with L-DOPA and MAO-inhibitors, Everett and Wiegand (1961) believe that dopamine plays a more important role than NE in regard to modulation of animal behavior (excitation or depression). On the other hand, Carlsson (1964) found that threo-dihydroxyphenylserine, which forms NE without the intermediate dopamine step, has central stimulant effects similar to those of DOPA. However, the latter finding could not be confirmed by others (Scheel-Krüger and Randrup, 1967; Aigner et al., 1968; Creveling et al., 1968).

γ) The Dopamine-hypothesis. Dopamine, which is the immediate precursor in the biosynthesis of NE has in all probability a role in brain different from that of NE. The distribution of dopamine differs from that of NE in that dopamine is particularly concentrated in certain nuclei of the extrapyramidal motor system. The highest dopamine content is found in the caudate nucleus and putamen (the corpus striatum), followed by the substantia nigra and the pars externa of the globus pallidus (Bertler and Rosengren, 1959; Sano et al., 1959; Ehringer and Hornykiewicz, 1960; Bertler, 1961; Hornykiewicz, 1963). This localization is so striking that a special role of dopamine in the extrapyramidal system must be assumed. This assumption has been corroborated by evidence that the dopamine content of the corpus striatum and substantia nigra is markedly diminished in human parkinsonism, a disease which mainly involves extrapyramidal centers (Ehringer and Hornykiewicz, 1960; Bernheimer et al., 1963; Hornykiewicz, 1963). If the lacking dopamine is replaced by injection of DOPA, akinesia (Birkmayer and Hornykiewicz, 1961, 1962, 1964) and rigor (Barbeau et al., 1962) are transiently diminished. Moreover, reserpine which reduces cerebral dopamine, and CPZ which affects dopamine metabolism in brain, (see chapter I, C, 5 c) cause clinical symptoms resembling parkinsonism. Destruction of certain nuclei of the extrapyramidal system also leads to disturbances of dopamine metabolism in the corpus striatum (Seitelberger et al., 1964; Andén et al., 1964 c; Poirier and Sourkes, 1965), indicating that the findings in human parkinsonism can be reproduced in animal experiments. All these findings represent strong arguments in favor of the hypothesis that dopamine is of great importance for the functioning of the extrapyramidal system. The role of dopamine for brain function is extensively discussed in the review of Hornykiewicz (1966 b).

b) Mechanism of Amine Release by Reserpine in CNS

Due to technical difficulties, the mechanism of amine release by reserpine in the CNS is not as well known as that in the periphery. However, it appears that as in the periphery, the central amine depletion is effected by inhibition of amine reuptake and binding.

Supporting this view is the finding of Green and Sawyer (1960) that in rat brain after reserpine treatment, bound NE decreases whereas the fraction containing free amine increases. As in the periphery, reserpine appears to indirectly inhibit the formation of NE from dopamine. This is corroborated by the observation that the NE concentration cannot be restored by administering MAO-inhibitors. Similar results have been obtained by Giarman and Schanberg (1958) who investigated the effect of reserpine on bound and free 5-HT in rat brain. Species differences may be involved as Weil-Malherbe and Bone (1959), Bertler et al. (1960) and Weil-Malherbe et al. (1961) have been unable to find differences in relative distribution of bound and free catecholamines in rabbit brain after reserpine injection. The possibility that reserpine blocks the uptake of newly synthesized 5-HT into the nerve cells of the CNS is given support by data of Kuntzman et al., (1956). This group noted that the 5-HTP-induced increase of 5-HT in brain does not occur in animals pretreated with reserpine.

The rate of amine release after intravenous reserpine injection is not the same for all amines. Dopamine and 5-HT are released at a faster rate than NE (see Bertler, 1961 b). This may be due to different turnover rates, since many studies indicate a faster turnover of 5-HT and dopamine in brain than of NE (Udenfriend et al., 1958; Holzer and Hornykiewicz, 1959; Carlsson et al., 1959 a).

After reserpine injection, the cerebral concentration of 3,4-dihydroxyphenylacetic acid, homovanillic acid and 5-hydroxyindoleacetic acid increases (Andén et al., 1963 b, 1964; Roos and Werdenius, 1964), indicating that greater amounts of dopamine and 5-HT undergo metabolic breakdown by O-methyltransferase and MAO than under normal conditions (compare also Rosengren, 1960). All these data corroborate the viewpoint that reserpine influences the storage and not the synthesis of dopamine and 5-HT.

c) Relationship between Amine Depletion and Central Reserpine Effects

It is impossible to discuss all the literature concerned with the relationship between cerebral amine depletion and central effects of reserpine. The most important results have recently been reviewed by Lewis (1963) and have also been mentioned in part in the preceding sections.

The fact that not only reserpine but also analogs, such as the benzoquinolizines, and structurally unrelated agents such as α-methyl-dopa and α-methyl-p-tyrosine, affect brain function in a characteristic manner attests to the existence of such a relationship. These agents share with reserpine the property of lowering the concentration of brain amines. Furthermore, the well known antagonism of reserpine by MAO-inhibitors is an additional indication of the connection between reserpine effect and amine depletion. Pretreatment with MAO-inhibitors not only blocks most peripheral and central reserpine effects but also prevents the release of brain amines.

It is more difficult, however, to relate some specific central reserpine effects to the decrease of a particular amine. As already mentioned, many investigators have associated the central depressant effect of reserpine with release of 5-HT, whereas others have emphasized the depletion of catecholamines. It appears to us that the most conclusive experimental evidence favors a connection between reserpine-induced extrapyramidal disturbances (parkinsonism) and changes in dopamine metabolism in brain.

Recently Feldberg and Myers (1963; 1964) have published data which suggest that 5-HT and NE in the hypothalamus may play an important role in the regulation of temperature. The impairment of heat regulation after reserpine (see this section, part 3 c) may be due to hypothalamic depletion of amines.

d) Other Biochemical Effects of Reserpine in CNS

Balzer et al. (1961 a) have observed that reserpine causes a long lasting reduction in the concentration of γ-aminobutyric acid (GABA) in brain of mice while concomitantly lowering the electroshock threshold. The increase in seizure susceptibility induced by reserpine (see this section, part 7 b) may be based on this biochemical finding. However, this can only be unequivocally determined when the functional significance of GABA in brain becomes known.

Abood and Romanchek (1957) have found that reserpine in large doses uncouples oxidative phosphorylation in rat mitochondria. This observation could not be confirmed by Lisovskaya and Livanova (cit. by Lewis, 1963). Kirpekar and Lewis (1959) noted a reduction in cerebral ATP content, whereas Balzer et al. (1961 b) have found no changes in ATP, ADP or AMP after reserpine administration. However, Balzer et al. (1961 b) have described an increase in lactic acid in brain following reserpine injection. The somewhat controversial findings make it unlikely that these biochemical changes represent the mechanism involved in the central effect of reserpine.

2. Effects on the Spinal Cord

According to Schneider et al. (1955 a), reserpine in i. v. doses of 5 mg/kg increases the patellar reflex in spinal cats. Monosynaptically transmitted potentials in the spinal cord are also enhanced. In contrast, some investigators have not been able to uncover an effect of reserpine on spinal reflex activity (Esplin and Heaton, 1957), whereas others have reported inhibition of mono- and polysynaptic potentials (Krivoy, 1957; Silvestrini and Maffii, 1959). These contradictory results may be explained by the recent observations (Roos and Steg, 1964; Steg, 1964) that reserpine rigidity in rats is coupled with increased excitability of α-motoneurons, inhibition of γ-fiber activity and enhanced monosynaptic reflexes. These authors believe that reserpine acts on supraspinal centers since the described effects do not occur in spinalized preparations. DOPA restores the reserpine-induced changes in spinal cord activity. Therefore it may be assumed that the enhancement of reflexes, after reserpine injection is due to dopamine depletion from extrapyramidal centers, possibly from the substantia nigra. The analogy to the rigidity of the parkinsonian patient is evident (compare this section, part 6 a, b).

3. Influence of Reserpine on Medullar, Meso- and Diencephalic Autonomic Functions

a) Antiemetic Effect

The antiemetic effect of reserpine is less specific than that of phenothiazine derivatives in that apomorphine emesis is only influenced by large doses of reserpine which already exert a marked sedative effect (Malthora and Sidhu, 1956).

b) Influence on Central Regulation of Circulation

There is no unanimous opinion in the literature on the question whether or not reserpine directly influences medullary or hypothalamic cardiovascular centers. In his review, Bein (1956) adduces arguments in favor of such a direct influence. Wang et al. (1964) (reference includes literature published after 1956) have not found evidence of a direct inhibitory effect of reserpine on these vascular regulatory regions. Several difficulties are met in this type of experiment: 1. Intravenous injection of reserpine is not suitable for uncovering potential central effects because of the marked effects of this alkaloid on the peripheral sympathetic system. 2. Experiments in which reserpine following peripheral or central administration exerts circulatory effects after a short latency (20—30 minutes) are to be interpreted with caution for it is known that the specific central effects of reserpine occur after a latency of 3—4 hours. 3. For the same reason, experiments carried out for only 1—2 hours after reserpine injection are insufficient to elucidate the problem of central versus peripheral effects of reserpine. Van Zwieten et al. (1966) have shown that 3—4 hours elapse before the carotid sinus reflex is significantly inhibited in cats after injection of small doses (up to 80 γ/kg) of reserpine into the vertebral artery. At this time brain catecholamines are maximally depleted whereas the NE-content of the heart remains unaltered. This makes a peripheral reserpine effect improbable in these experiments. The same investigators also demonstrated that reserpine selectively diminishes the chemo-receptor reflex. Since, according to Bein (1955), reserpine does not have a direct effect on the chemoreceptors themselves, one has to assume that the diminution of the reflex is effected by a central depressant action. This interpretation is in agreement with the fact that the respiratory depression induced by reserpine, and observed in every species, is mediated by an effect on those brain regions which respond to afferent impulses from chemoreceptors (Bein, 1956).

c) Influence on Body Temperature and Appetite

Reserpine lowers the body temperature of mice, rats, guinea pigs, cats, dogs and monkeys (for reference, see Bein, 1956). This appears to be due to an impairment of temperature regulating centers. In high environmental temperature reserpine may increase body temperature. In man the hypothermic effect of reserpine is insignificant. In contrast to CPZ, reserpine does not possess an antipyretic effect; in rabbits, fever induced by pyrogens is not lowered by reserpine (Bein et al., 1953).

The hypothesis that NE and 5-HT play a role in temperature regulation (Feldberg and Myers, 1963, 1964) is important in regard to the reserpine effect on temperature regulating centers. If Feldberg and Myers are correct in assuming that changes in amine concentration alter the function of these centers, it is justifiable to postulate that reserpine inactivates the hypothalamic temperature regulating mechanisms by reducing the catecholamine and 5-HT concentration in the corresponding brain areas.

Appetite, also regulated by the hypothalamus, is enhanced by reserpine (as well as by phenothiazines). Therefore, chronic reserpine treatment often increases body weight.

d) Influence on Central Sympathetic Mechanisms

Sham rage in decerebrated cats, elicited by the slightest nociceptive stimuli and accompanied by the activation of the central and peripheral sympathetic system, is diminished by reserpine but cannot be completely suppressed (Schneider et al., 1955).

Iggo and Vogt (1960) examined the question of whether or not reserpine influences the central sympathetic outflow by recording spontaneous preganglionic action potentials in the cervical sympathetic nerve of cats. No changes of impulse traffic after reserpine pretreatment could be detected by these authors. In contrast, Bein (1955) has noted a complete suppression of electrical activity in sympathetic cardiac nerves after reserpine administration. (Compare also with this chapter, section c, 1 a, β.)

4. Influence on Electrophysiologic Manifestations in Brain

a) EEG Changes

Numerous investigations are concerned with the effects of reserpine on the EEG in man and several animal species. (The literature is discussed in extenso by Lewis, 1963.)

The spontaneous human EEG is not altered by therapeutic doses of reserpine (Monroe et al., 1955; Arellano and Jeri, 1956; Dennison et al., 1955; Hafkenschiel et al., 1955). Similarly, no significant EEG alterations are found in monkeys (Schneider and Earl, 1954) or in cats (Killam and Killam, 1957). The absence of significant EEG changes is in sharp contrast to the marked sedative effect of reserpine. In cats, reserpine does not change the threshold and duration of the EEG and behavioral arousal reaction induced by direct stimulation of the reticular formation (Killam and Killam, 1957).

According to Barraclough (1955), reserpine is also devoid of an effect on the threshold response to mesencephalic stimulation in rats. However, in monkeys the threshold is raised for EEG and behavioral arousal by direct stimulation of the reticular formation (Takaori and Deneau, 1962). Rabbits appear to be particularly sensitive to reserpine. Thus, Gangloff and Monnier (1955) reported that the threshold for cortical and diencephalic stimulation was increased and that thalamic and cortical spike discharges induced by low frequency stimulation of the ponto-bulbar reticular formation were suppressed by reserpine. Moreover, a shift towards high frequency and low amplitude occurs in the electrocorticogram of rabbits approximately

30 minutes after reserpine injection (Rinaldi and Himwich, 1955 a, b; Gangloff and Monnier, 1955; Kikuchi, 1961; Sailer and Stumpf, 1957). This activation is believed to be due to stimulation of the ascending reticular formation (Rinaldi and Himwich, 1955 a, b), an assumption corroborated by the observation that transection at the level of the superior colliculi abolishes the EEG-arousal reaction (Sailer and Stumpf, 1957). These investigators have also found that reserpine obliterates the arousal reaction induced by mescaline or LSD. This antagonism must take place anterior to the colliculi since the EEG effects of mescaline and LSD are not depressed after transection of the mesencephalon. In contrast to the above mentioned results that reserpine induces an arousal pattern in the electrocorticogram, Kikuchi (1961) claims that the EEG arousal is diminished in unanesthetized rabbits following reserpine.

Recently, Himwich and coworkers (Pscheidt et al., 1964) have reinvestigated the effects of reserpine on the rabbit EEG. They have found that it is relevant whether reserpine is administered before the surgical intervention (implantation of electrodes) or afterwards. The EEG arousal, which lasts for several hours when reserpine is injected after the operative procedures, is considered to be an artifact. In rabbits receiving reserpine before the operation, EEG-activation is observed 30—60 minutes after injection followed 5 hours later by the typical pattern of sedation. The investigators postulate a dual action: the initial activation phase due to liberation of catecholamines and 5-HT by reserpine, followed by a phase of amine depletion coupled with sedation during which even painful stimuli are ineffective in eliciting an EEG-arousal reaction.

b) Influence on the Thalamic Projection Systems

Several reports exist on the influence of reserpine on specific nuclei of the thalamus. Gangloff and Monnier (1957) have noted an increase in threshold for afterdischarges in the lateral thalamus, without change in duration, after doses of up to 2 mg/kg of reserpine in unanesthetized rabbits. In monkeys, reserpine lowered the threshold for after-discharges induced by stimulation of the anterior dorsal nucleus (Delgado and Mihailovic, 1956).

Results on the influence of reserpine on the diffuse thalamic projection system are contradictory. In rabbit, 1.5 mg/kg of reserpine initially enhances the thalamocortical recruiting response, followed by a diminution 1—2 hours after administration of reserpine (Gangloff and Monnier, 1957). In unanesthetized rabbits, no effect or a slight depression of the recruiting response has been noted (Kikuchi, 1961). According to Killam and Killam (1956), as well as Sigg and Schneider (1957), thalamocortical recruiting responses in cats are not altered by reserpine.

c) Influence on the Limbic System

Several investigators believe that reserpine has no significant influence on the functions of the limbic system. Thus, Monroe et al. (1955) have been unable to uncover an effect of reserpine on the spontaneous electrical activity of the amygdaloid nucleus and hippocampus in schizophrenic patients during acute and chronic treatment. Reserpine also seems to be devoid of any effect on the limbic system in monkey (Delgado and Mihailovic, 1956; Takaori and Deneau, 1962 a).

On the other hand, MacLean et al. (1955—56) describe slow wave activity in the hippocampus of the cat after reserpine injection similar to the effects of local application of carbachol. The effects of reserpine and topically applied carbachol are also similar in regard to general behavior and conditioned reflexes. Gangloff and Monnier (1957) noticed convulsive spikes in the limbic system of rabbits after administration of larger doses of reserpine, while the threshold for after-discharges was unaltered but their duration was somewhat prolonged. Killam et al. (1957) made similar observations. In cats chronically treated with reserpine the threshold is lowered, and spontaneous spiking occurs in the hippocampus (Killam and Killam, 1957). According to Sigg and Schneider (1957), 1 mg/kg of reserpine prolongs after-discharges elicited by amygdaloid and hippocampal stimulation in spinal cats. However, some of these positive results are disputed, e. g., Hamel and Kaelber (1961) decidedly contest the observations of MacLean et al. (1955, 1956) and Killam and Killam (1956).

If the evidence for an effect of reserpine on the limbic system is accepted, it is obvious to relate it to a depletion of 5-HT (and catecholamines?) found in relatively high concentrations in this brain region. However, a connection between electrophysiological phenomena and the physiological significance of 5-HT in this area cannot be established with certainty yet.

d) Effects on Cortex

Most investigators have found no significant effects of small doses of reserpine on cortex (Schneider et al., 1955 a; Delgado and Mihailovic, 1956; Takaori and Deneau, 1962 a; Bein, 1955). Large doses (up to 2 mg/kg) increase the threshold for cortical after-discharges without changing their duration (Gangloff and Monnier, 1955).

5. Influence of Reserpine on Behavior

a) Effect on General Behavior

The most conspicuous central effect of reserpine is sedation and decrease in motor activity occurring in many species (for literature reference, see Bein, 1956). The type of sedation is somewhat similar to that seen after phenothiazines and differs from that seen as a result of administration of hypnotics and general anesthetics. Even after very large doses, hypnosis does not occur. The animals can be aroused at all times from their apathy by external stimuli but will resume the sleep-like state soon after termination of the stimulus. Under the influence of reserpine, cats and dogs often take up their natural sleeping position after displaying the typical behavior which precedes sleep. Chusid et al. (1955) and particularly Cole and Glees (1956) described a peculiar "fetal" position and marked tremor in monkeys (Macaca mulatta, Macaca nemestrina) after i. v. injection of 1—1.5 mg/kg of reserpine. The animals can be placed in unnatural positions which are not spontaneously corrected. Similar to bulbocapnine catelepsy, the animals retain food in their mouth without consuming it and exhibit increased grasping reflexes characteristic of toxic catalepsy. Reserpine-catalepsy can also be demonstrated in several other species. The "taming" effect of reserpine is equally typical and is particularly obvious in aggressive monkeys (Chusid et al., 1955; Plummer et al., 1954; Weiskrantz and Wilson, 1955). Inhibition of sham rage by reserpine has already been mentioned.

The effect of reserpine in man has been examined with a battery of psychologic tests by Lehmann and Csank (1957). In contrast to CPZ, reserpine enhances the sensitivity to after-images. Watt and Crookes (1961) conclude from their investigations on manic female patients that reserpine inhibits visual inflow, whereas, in contrast to CPZ, motor and associative functions remain uninfluenced.

b) Influence on Conditioned Behavior

The methods of inducing conditioned behavior by training and the difficulty in interpreting the findings obtained by such manipulations have already been discussed in the chapter on phenothiazines (chapter I, section C, 4 b). From the literature, it is concluded that reserpine inhibits conditioned behavior in every species examined. A more detailed discussion is found in publications by Jacobsen (1959), and Dews and Morse (1961). The avoidance-escape response is diminished but rarely completely suppressed in rats, dogs and monkeys. In all procedures investigated, reserpine also obliterates the motivation for obtaining a reward (Brady, 1956). Utilizing the self-stimulation technique of Olds (1958), with implanted electrodes in the hypothalamus and nucleus amygdalae, a reduction in bar pressing has been observed after reserpine injection similar to the effect obtained with CPZ (Olds et al., 1956; see also chapter I, section C, 4 b). Sometimes these effects were absent (Olds et al., 1957).

The reserpine-induced suppression of the conditioned avoidance response in mice and cats can be restored by injection of L-DOPA. The DOPA-effect parallels the recovery of cerebral dopamine levels and is not related to the restoration of the NE-content (Seiden and Carlsson, 1963, 1964; Seiden and Hanson, 1964). Since inhibition of the conditioned avoidance response by reserpine and phenothiazines may be at least partly due to an influence of these agents on extra-pyramidal centers (vide chapter I), these findings would represent another example of the evidence that the extrapyramidal effects of reserpine are antagonized by L-DOPA. This is in agreement with other experiments (see this chapter and section, part 6 b) indicating the importance of brain dopamine for the functioning of the extrapyramidal centers. However, it should be stressed that the above mentioned experiments with L-DOPA do not necessarily explain the mechanism by which reserpine exerts its central depressant effect. It is even uncertain that changes in conditioned behavior relate directly to depletion of brain amines. Thus, Weissman and Finger (1962) have found that only one of the two reserpine-like benzoquinolizines which inhibit the conditioned avoidance response releases brain amines. Even less evidence exists for a relationship between amine depletion induced by reserpine and its therapeutic effect in psychoses. At present, only the extrapyramidal symptomatology caused by reserpine can be, with reasonable certainty, related to the amine (dopamine) depleting effect of this drug (see below).

6. Extrapyramidal Motor Disturbances in Man and Catalepsy in Animals

a) Parkinson Syndrome in Man and Catalepsy in Animals

As early as the first Indian investigations on the clinical effects of rauwolfia extracts, the occurrence of reversible extrapyramidal symptoms are mentioned. Reserpine can cause a parkinson-like syndrome similar to that induced by phenothiazines. The susceptibility of individual patients to this reserpine side-effect varies greatly. In most cases, parkinson-like symptoms occur if the daily doses of reserpine reach 2 mg. Those patients who are sensitive to phenothiazines are also susceptible to reserpine. A combination of both drugs leads particularly often to parkinsonism. After cessation of reserpine therapy, the extrapyramidal symptoms disappear spontaneously, though often very slowly.

The parkinson-like effects, particularly the marked akinesia, make it understandable that reserpine also suppresses the hyperkinesia in Huntington's Chorea, sometimes leading to a complete motor immobilization of the patient.

Mice, rats, rabbits, cats and monkeys (for literature reference, see Stumpf, 1962; Zetler et al., 1960) exhibit catalepsy after reserpine administration. The experiments of Chusid et al. (1955) have already been mentioned in which 1 mg/kg i. v. of reserpine caused coarse tremors, hyperkinesia, a semistuporous state and inability to correct imposed unnatural postures. Moreover, Cole and Glees (1956) have described a typical sign of catalepsy in which monkeys (Macaca mulatta and Macaca nemestrina) are unable to chew and swallow food which was put in their mouth.

b) Mechanism Involved in the Extrapyramidal Effects of Reserpine

It has already been emphasized that of all central reserpine effects the influence on extrapyramidal centers is best documented biochemically (see also review by Curzon, 1968). This is based on the hypothesis of dopamine's significance in the function of these centers (vide this chapter, section 3, C 1, γ). There is a satisfactory biochemical correlation between human parkinsonism (particularly postencephalic parkinsonism) and reserpine-induced parkinsonism. In animal experiments reserpine depletes extrapyramidal nuclei (nucleus caudatus and putamen [= corpus striatum] and probably the substantia nigra of their dopamine. Hornykiewicz and colleagues have demonstrated that there is a lack of dopamine in the same brain areas of patients with genuine parkinsonism (see Hornykiewicz, 1964 d). Increase of brain dopamine by injection of L-DOPA, the dopamine precursor which penetrates the blood-brain barrier, diminishes akinesia and rigidity of reserpine-parkinsonism (Degkwitz et al., 1960) and of the genuine parkinson syndrome as well (Birkmayer and Hornykiewicz, 1961, 1962, 1964; Barbeau et al., 1962; Gerstenbrand and Pateisky, 1962; Gerstenbrand et al., 1963; Friedhoff et al., 1963; Hirschmann and Mayer, 1964; Umbach and Baumann, 1964). This therapeutic effect of L-DOPA is enhanced and prolonged by MAO-inhibitors which themselves possess only weak and somewhat inconsistent activity in this respect. The striking analogy between the rigor of the parkinson syndrome and reserpine-parkinsonism has also been observed by Roos and Steg (1964) using electrophysiological methods (see also Steg, 1964). In both states a marked increase in excitability of α-motoneurons coupled with inhibition of γ-fiber activity is observed. The reserpine effect is believed to be supraspinal in origin. Birkmayer and Hornykiewicz (1964) conclude that the morphological substrates may be the neurons of the substantia nigra. In support of this view, these authors state that severe parkinsonism is less aggravated by reserpine than mild forms of parkinsonism. Since the severity of parkinsonism is proportional to the extent of destruction in the substantia nigra, which, according to Hassler (1953), is the anatomical substrate of parkinsonism, it can be assumed that the extrapyramidal effects of reserpine are dependent on the intactness of neurons in the substantia nigra. On the other hand, the intactness of the corpus striatum is not a prerequisite for the development of reserpine-parkinsonism. In spite of the fact that in Huntington's Chorea the corpus striatum is injured by degeneration of the majority of the small neuron cells, reserpine still elicits the parkinson syndrome, probably since the substantia nigra is undamaged in this disease.

Himwich and Rinaldi (1957) proposed that the extrapyramidal effects of reserpine and CPZ are due to an uncoordinated hyperactivity in the descending reticular formation. This hypothesis is based on the older finding that reserpine stimulates the ascending system of the reticular formation (see this chapter, section C, 4 a). In reexamining his initial experiments, Himwich found, however, that reserpine elicits only a shortlasting stimulation of the reticular formation followed by a longer-lasting depression (Pscheidt et al., 1964).

Therefore, it can be assumed that the extrapyramidal symptoms are primarily caused by a depression of certain brain stem areas (e. g., substantia nigra). This depression may be the consequence of transmitter depletion from dopaminergic neurons in the substantia nigra, analogous to the genuine parkinson syndrome.

7. Interactions of Reserpine with other Centrally Active Agents

a) Central Depressants

The specific pharmacological property of a central depressant agent determines the type of interaction with reserpine. The hypnotic effect of barbiturates (Brodie et al., 1955; Cronheim and Toekes, 1955; Slater et al., 1955) and alcohol (Brodie et al., 1955) is prolonged by reserpine. In contrast, the anticonvulsive effect of barbiturates, diphenylhydantoin or mephenesin is diminished (Chen and Ensor, 1954). The analgesic effect of morphine (Schneider, 1954; Schaumann, 1958), pethidine and codeine (Sigg et al., 1958) is also reduced by reserpine.

Possibly there is a relationship between 5-HT liberation by reserpine and prolongation of sleeping time. Holtz et al. (1957) found that reserpine-induced prolongation of hexobarbital-sleeping time is shortened when 5-HT is administered simultaneously. This is difficult to reconcile with the observation that 5-HT, 5-HTP, tryptophan and tryptamine, per se, prolong hexobarbital hypnosis, while dopamine and DOPA are devoid of such an effect. Barbiturates are claimed to increase 5-HT in brain (Anderson and Bonnycastle, 1960), a finding which Efron and Gessa (1963) have not been able to confirm.

The central depressant effect of reserpine is transiently antagonized by amphetamine, methamphetamine, methylphenidate or L-DOPA (compare e. g., Tripod et al., 1954; Cole and Glees, 1956; Everett et al., 1957; Carlsson et al., 1957a; Kobinger, 1958a; Blaschko and Chrusciel, 1960; Degkwitz et al., 1960).

b) Central Stimulants, Electroshock and Convulsants

In mice, reserpine inhibits psychomotor stimulation induced by caffeine, scopolamine, morphine and cocaine. However, amphetamine-induced hyperkinesia is apparently not antagonized by reserpine (Tripod et al., 1954, Kobinger, 1958 a) but rather potentiated (Smith, 1963). Nevertheless, reserpine appears to offer some protection against lethal doses of amphetamine (Cronheim and Toekes, 1955).

The Straub-tail phenomenon is antagonized by reserpine (Tripod et al., 1954).

The convulsant effects of strychnine, picrotoxin or nicotine cannot be prevented by reserpine (Tripod et al., 1954). Reserpine even enhances the convulsant effects of caffeine and pentylenetetrazol (Chen et al., 1954; Bianchi, 1956; Sacra and McColl, 1958; Hertting, 1958, Kobinger, 1958 b). The threshold for tonic extensor spasms induced by electroshock is significantly lowered by reserpine (Chen and Ensor 1954; Chen et al., 1954; Jenney, 1954; Everett et al., 1955; Slater et al., 1955). The susceptibility to seizures induced by reserpine is somewhat diminished by anticonvulsants (Chen and Ensor, 1954). However, as has already been mentioned, reserpine antagonizes the anticonvulsant effects of these agents. A possible relationship between the convulsant effect of reserpine and a diminution of GABA-content in brain has already been discussed (Balzer et al., 1961 a; see also this chapter, section C, 1 d). Most of these central reserpine effects can be antagonized by MAO-inhibitors (see chapter V, section C, 1 e, 2 a, E).

D. Endocrine Effects of Reserpine

Gaunt et al. (1954) were the first to examine a potential influence of reserpine on endocrine glands (for a discussion, see Gaunt et al., 1961). Reserpine causes a hypertrophy of the adrenal cortex (Gaunt et al., 1954; Hertting and Hornykiewicz, 1957). It depletes the adrenal gland of ascorbic acid (Saffran and Vogt, 1960; Brodie et al., 1961 a) and increases plasma corticosterone (Brodie et al., 1961 a). All these effects are the consequence of ACTH-release from the anterior pituitary (Kitay et al., 1959; Saffran and Vogt, 1960; Westermann et al., 1960). This is corroborated by the finding that injection of cortisone, which diminishes ACTH-release by negative feedback, inhibits reserpine-induced hypertrophy of the adrenal cortex (Hertting and Hornykiewicz, 1957). Hypophysectomy also abolishes this reserpine effect (Brodie et al., 1961 a). The same authors have demonstrated that reserpine analogs with a sedative component, such as raunescine and rescinnamine, affect the pituitary-adrenal axis in the same manner as reserpine, whereas derivatives lacking a CNS-depressant effect (isoreserpine, isoraunescine and serpentine) are devoid of such action. Opinions on the mechanism of ACTH-release by reserpine differ: Gaunt et al. (1954, 1961) and Saffran and Vogt (1960) regard it as consequence of unspecific "stress", whereas Brodie et al. (1961 a) and Westermann (1965) believe it to be a specific influence of reserpine on the hypothalamic-pituitary system. The fact that reserpine pretreated rats do not develop a typical "stress" response to pain, cold or an acute injection of reserpine is interpreted by Westermann (1961) as a consequence of ACTH-depletion of the pituitary by reserpine. Plasma 17-hydroxycorticosteroid concentration is increased by reserpine in animals (Egdahl et al., 1956; Harwood and Mason, 1957) and man (Tui et al., 1956). These findings are also in agreement with the occurrence of ACTH-release by reserpine.

Secretion of gonadotropin from the anterior pituitary is inhibited by reserpine with the consequence of arresting estrus and menstruation (De Feo and Reynalds, 1956). Fertility is decreased and the decidual reaction of the uterus is modified (Gaunt et al., 1954; Tuchmann-Duplessis and Mercier-Parot, 1956; De Feo, 1957). During menopause, urine excretion of gonadotropin is diminished in women treated with reserpine (Khazan et al., 1960). On the other hand, secretion of luteotropin from the anterior pituitary is enhanced by reserpine (and chlorpromazine). Barraclough and Sawyer (1959) have found that a single injection of reserpine induces pseudopregnancy in rats with the corresponding decidual changes in the uterus. After chronic treatment, a number of large corpora lutea develop in the ovaries. These authors believe that stimulation of luteotropin secretion is related to the depressant effect of reserpine (and CPZ) on the hypothalamus.

Reserpine also stimulates prolactin secretion, leading to galactorrhea in animals and women (for literature reference see Barraclough and Sawyer, 1959; Gaunt et al., 1961).

In adult male rats reserpine (in doses of up to 0.5 mg/kg for 2—6 weeks) causes atrophy of testicles, prostate and seminal vesicles, whereas smaller doses have no adverse effects in this respect (Khazan et al., 1960). Male patients may complain of diminished libido (Wilkins, 1954).

According to Moon and Turner (1959), thyrotropic hormone production is also inhibited. However, the thyroid uptake of [131]iodine is not affected (Goodman et al., 1955; compare contradictory results of Mayer et al., 1956), whereas the release of ^{131}I and thyroxin from the thyroid gland appears to be inhibited (Moon and Turner, 1959). Reserpine exerts a beneficial influence on cardiovascular disorders (tachycardia) in thyrotoxicosis. It is possible that this effect is related to the central inhibition or to the suppression of the peripheral adrenergic nervous system.

It is noteworthy that treatment of newly captured wild rabbits with reserpine prevents the hyperthyroid response, the suppression of spermiogenesis and those morphologic changes in hypothalamus and hypophysis which develop as a result of captivity (Miline et al., 1957). This effect may also be central (hypothalamic?) in nature.

In water- and sodium chloride-loaded rats, reserpine exerts an acute antidiuretic effect (Gaunt et al., 1954; Meier et al., 1955). However, the urinary excretion of sodium and potassium in dog and man is not altered by reserpine (Bein, 1956).

E. Metabolic Fate of Reserpine

The metabolic fate of reserpine in animals has been investigated by Bein (1956), Maynert and Plummer et al. (1957). Several metabolic pathways seem to exist. Hydrolysis leads to methylreserpate and 3,4,5-trimethoxybenzoate. Reserpic acid, syringic acid and syringoyl-methyl-reserpate have also been found. O-methylation also appears to be possible.

Sheppard et al. (1955) have studied the tissue distribution of reserpine in animals. Immediately after injection the highest concentrations of reserpine are found in spleen, liver and kidney. Several hours after administration, when other tissues begin to contain less reserpine, an accumulation in fat tissue takes place. A preferential storage in brain does not occur, even after centrally active doses of reserpine. Originally, it had been accepted with certainty that reserpine can only be detected for a few hours in brain. However, Sheppard et al. (1955) were able to detect small amounts of ^{3}H-labelled reserpine as long as 48 hours after administration. Contrary to previous viewpoints, one therefore has to assume that minute amounts of reserpine are present during the whole duration of its central action. Unfortunately, it has not been possible to correlate brain concentration of reserpine with the degree of its central actions, e. g., sedation.

F. Adverse Reactions and Dangers

1. Suicide and Fatal Poisoning

Successful suicide and poisoning with lethal outcome due to reserpine or reserpine-like agents, have not been reported. Overdosing leads to profound somnolence and long lasting hypotension. Extrapyramidal disturbances are also observed.

2. Central Nervous System

Dysfunctions of the extrapyramidal system have already been discussed (see this chapter, section C, 6 a). In contrast to CPZ, typical dystonias are generally not observed during reserpine treatment. The patients often exhibit the classical signs of parkinsonism with tremor, rigor and akinesia as principal symptoms. These disturbances may last for several months after termination of treatment and may even be irreversible (Uhrbrand and Faurbye, 1960).

Similar to phenothiazines, reserpine can cause depression. This side-effect of reserpine is more frequent and more severe than the phenothiazine depression representing one of the causes of the not infrequent attempts of suicide. Inner restlessness, insomnia and delirium may occur. Occasionally epileptiform convulsions are observed during reserpine treatment. This side-effect is probably related to the property of reserpine to lower the convulsive threshold for numerous convulsants and electroshock (see this chapter, section C, 7 b). In patients with brain damage, hyperpyrexia, paralysis of ocular muscles and decerebrate states can be precipitated by reserpine. Sometimes a choreo-athetotic syndrome develops (Hollister, 1957).

3. Autonomic Nervous System

Disturbances of the autonomic nervous system manifest themselves in diminished sympathetic and enhanced parasympathetic activity. The following symptoms are relatively frequent: bradycardia, hypotension and susceptibility to collapse, nasal congestion, increased salivation, diarrhea, stomach ulcers, hematemesis and melena. The occurrence of cardiac arrhythmias has repeatedly been reported, particularly after simultaneous administration of digitalis preparations (Hollister, 1964). Withrington and Zaimis (1961) have found that 1 mg/kg of reserpine severely damages the heart muscle in cats.

4. Miscellaneous Side-effects

In contrast to phenothiazines, reserpine does not cause jaundice or bone marrow abnormalities. A few cases of thrombopenic purpura have been reported (see Domino, 1962 b). Proof of allergic reactions to reserpine has not been established.

The diverse effects of reserpine on endocrine glands have already been discussed (see this chapter, section D). Reserpine can cause a marked body weight gain which is due partly to an increase in appetite and partly to fluid retention with the formation of edema.

IV. Minor Tranquilizers

Minor tranquilizers are distinctly different from either the rauwolfia alkaloids or the phenothiazines in that they are not effective in the treatment of psychoses. In contrast to the neuroleptic agents, minor tranquilizers exert little effect on the peripheral autonomic nervous system and do not, as a rule, produce extrapyramidal effects. They are distinguished by their anticonvulsant properties and their depressant affects on spinal reflex activity. The most widely used representatives of this class of compounds are meprobamate, chlordiazepoxide and diazepam.

Pertinent reviews on the pharmacology of meprobamate have been written by Berger (1954) and on the benzodiazepines, chlordiazepoxide and diazepam, by Randall et al. (1961), and by Zbinden (1967).

A. Central Effects

1. Behavioral Effects

The benzodiazepine tranquilizers reduce aggressive behavior in monkeys (Randall et al., 1960, 1961) whereas meprobamate has only a slight taming effect. Isolation-induced fighting in mice is abolished by chlordiazepoxide, less so by meprobamate (Scriabine and Blake, 1962; Cole and Wolf, 1966). Minor tranquilizers also inhibit the irritability of rats with lesions in the septum (Hunt, 1957; Raitt et al., 1961; Schallek et al., 1962). This effect is also seen, however, after administration of phenothiazines (Stark and Henderson, 1966).

In general, the minor tranquilizers markedly increase the rate of occurrence of previously suppressed behavior (Geller and Seifter, 1960; see also discussion by Margoles and Stein, 1967). In rats and squirrel monkeys submitted to the continuous avoidance procedure small doses of chlordiazepoxide or diazepam cause avoidance failure as indicated by the increase in shock rate, whereas meprobamate causes loss of both avoidance and escape responses indicative of the inability to respond (Heise and Boff, 1962). In conflict situations in which a conditioned lever-pressing response in rats is rewarded with food and simultaneously punished with shock, the benzodiazepine tranquilizers as well as meprobamate attenuate the conflict behavior as indicated by continued lever pressing during the conditioning stimulus (Geller et al., 1962). In other models of experimental neurosis, benzodiazepines have also been shown to attenuate passive avoidance responses. The consequences of more general stressful situations, such as the occurrence of ulcers by the restraining of rats, can be diminished by chlordiazepoxide (Haot et al., 1964). The increase in plasma of free fatty acids induced by repeated electroshock is also significantly reduced by benzodiazepines and meprobamate. However, this response is not restricted to these compounds since rauwolfia alkaloids and phenothiazines are also active (Khan et al., 1964).

2. Studies of Electrophysiological Events in the CNS

Minor tranquilizers tend to shift the frequency spectrum of the electrocorticogram towards the slow side, particularly if an activation pattern exists prior to administration. It is generally assumed that the minor tranquilizers act predominantly on subcortical areas. The limbic system seems to be particularly sensitive and a significant slowing in the electrical activity of the septum, hippocampus and the amygdala has been shown for chlordiazepoxide and, in part, for meprobamate (Kletzkin and Swan, 1959; Randall et al., 1961; Schallek et al., 1962). Not only is spontaneous activity in the hippocampus slowed by chlordiazepoxide and diazepam (Arrigo et al., 1965), but the hippocampal response to amygdaloid stimulation is also depressed (Morillo et al., 1962). Moreover, all three minor tranquilizers shorten the electrical after-discharges in the limbic system (Kletzkin and Berger, 1959; Schallek et al., 1962; Horovitz et al., 1963; Requin et al., 1963). Seizures induced chemically by implanting acetylcholine into the amygdala are blocked by diazepam (Hernández-Peón et al., 1964). Some investigators have also found changes in the seizure activity of the cerebral cortex. Thus the threshold for initiating convulsant paroxysms by electrical stimulation of the cortex is raised (Roldan and Escobar, 1961) and after-discharges in the cortex have been noted to be diminished by chlordiazepoxide and meprobamate. High doses of chlordiazepoxide also abolish the epileptiform-discharges in monkeys induced by topical application of alumina cream (Chusid and Kopeloff, 1962). These electrophysiological results are corroborated by the observation of appropriate reduction of behavioral responses to electrical stimulation in various brain regions (Arrigo et al., 1965; Kido and Yamamoto, 1965).

The electrocortical arousal response elicited by mesencephalic reticular stimulation or sensory stimulation is diminished by meprobamate and benzodiazepines given in relatively large doses (Monnier and Graber, 1962). However, there is no significant change in the thalamocortical recruiting responses. Autonomic responses elicited by hypothalamic stimulation (e. g. vasopressor effect) are blocked by benzodiazepines (Schallek et al., 1964), indicating interference with central autonomic activity.

An interesting and apparently specific effect of barbiturates and meprobamate on the bioelectrical activity of the nucleus ruber in rabbits has been described by Schimmerl and Stumpf (1958). These two drugs induce a regular rythm of 4 pulses per second (pps) which gradually increases to 20 pps.

3. Anticonvulsant Effects

As is evident from the electrophysiological investigations (see section A, 2), the minor tranquilizers have marked anticonvulsant properties. Whereas the seizures induced by maximal electroshock and strychnine are diminished only after doses already causing muscle-relaxant effects, pentamethylenetetrazole-induced convulsions are antagonized by very low doses of chlordiazepoxide and diazepam (Randall et al., 1960; Bastian, 1961; Lanoir et al., 1965). Benzodiazepines also effectively block cocaine-induced seizures in rats in contrast to diphenylhydantoin and phenobarbital which are ineffective in this respect (Eidelberg et al., 1965), The high sensitivity of pentamethylenetetrazol-induced seizures to benzodiazepines and meprobamate are reminiscent of the activity spectrum of trimethadione (Goodman et al., 1946).

4. Effects on the Spinal Cord

The disruption of coordinate motor behavior which is observed particularly with chlordiazepoxide, diazepam and, to a lesser extent, meprobamate may be due to the marked muscle relaxant effect of these compounds (Randall, 1960; Randall et al., 1960; Klupp and Kähling, 1965; Gluckman, 1965). All three minor tranquilizers diminish polysynaptic reflexes, e. g., crossed extensor and flexor reflexes in spinal and decerebrated cats (Hendly et al., 1954; Wilson and Talbot, 1960; Randall et al., 1961). The muscle relaxant effect of benzodiazepines is particularly pronounced in the decerebrate animal (Tardieu et al., 1964; Jimenez-Pabon and Nelson, 1965; Schallek, 1966; Ngai et al., 1966). Since the benzodiazepines are considerably more active in the decerebrate than in the spinal preparation, an action on supraspinal controls of reflex activity has to be assumed. Recent evidence also indicates that the reflex depressant effect of diazepam stems chiefly from an intensification and prolongation of presynaptic inhibition of proprio- and extero ceptive afferents in the spinal cord (Schmidt et al., 1967).

5. Biochemical Effects

In contrast to neuroleptic agents (phenothiazines, butyrophenones, reserpine) the tranquilizers do not significantly change the cerebral metabolism of catecholamines *in vivo* (Laverty and Sharman, 1965; Roos 1965; Da Prada and Pletscher, 1966). Moreover, tranquilizers, unlike antipsychotic agents, have little effect on the spontaneous release of epinephrine from adrenal medullary granules or the 5-HT outflow from blood platelets (Pletscher et al., 1967).

B. Peripheral Effects

Neither meprobamate nor the benzodiazepines possess any significant peripheral pharmacological properties. This distinguishes these compounds from the neuroleptics, the MAO-inhibitors and tricyclic antidepressants.

C. Metabolic Studies

C^{14}-labelled meprobamate is equally distributed in the body. Ten to 20% of the drug is excreted unchanged in urine (Agronoff et al., 1957). Two metabolites are the result of the oxidation of the methyl and propyl groups. Two other metabolic products are glucuronic acid conjugates; their acid hydrolysis yields the hydroxymethyl-derivative of meprobamate (Walkenstein et al., 1958).

The benzodiazepines are metabolized similarly in dog and man, but differently in other species, e. g rats. Chlordiazepoxide is first demethylated, then deaminated to the lactam (Koechlin et al., 1965). While ring opening subsequently occurs in the first breakdown of the lactam, this does not take place with diazepam, which is first demethylated and then hydroxylated in the three position. The demethylated hydroxylated product is oxazepam which is excreted as glucuronide (Schwartz et al., 1965).

D. Adverse Reactions

The side-effects of meprobamate and benzodiazepines are characteristically coupled to the CNS-depressant and muscle-relaxant properties. Drowsiness, lethargy and ataxia are the most common symptoms (Hollister, 1961). Elderly patients are particularly sensitive, and in severe poisoning or suicide attempts coma and hypotension may occur. Because of the weak effect of minor tranquilizers on the autonomic system, cardio-vascular and respiratory abnormalities are minor even after large doses. Hepatotoxic and nephrotoxic effects are absent. Impairment of sexual function, headache, nausea and idiosyncrasy to these drugs have been sporadically noted. Similar to barbiturates benzodiazepines and meprobamate may induce a peculiar hyperexcitability and irritability. Hyperactivity in rodents and monkeys has been observed particularly in doses below those inducing CNS-depression (Sternbach et al., 1964; Randall et al., 1965). An undesirable side-effect seen both in animals and man may be stimulation of appetite with a resulting weight gain (Randall, 1960).

Benzodiazepines as well as meprobamate enhance the CNS-depressant effects of various agents, e. g., phenothiazines, barbiturates and non-barbiturate-hypnotics to some extent (Zbinden et al., 1961; Frommel et al., 1963). A combination of these drugs has therefore to be approached cautiously. There seems to be no additive effect with morphine and meperidine (Frommel et al., 1964; Sadove et al., 1965). In animals chlordiazepoxide and diazepam do not have an effect on the rate of metabolic destruction of ethyl alcohol, a finding which has been confirmed in man.

Controversal accounts are found in the literature in regard to the compulsive use of and physical dependence on minor tranquilizers (for reviews see Zbinden and Randall, 1967). It is however, established that withdrawal symptoms may occur when chronic administration of large doses is abruptly terminated. Seizures, coma, aggravation of the psychopathological state, insomnia and excitatory states have been observed (Hollister and Glazener, 1960; Hollister et al., 1961; for critical reviews see Zbinden and Randall, 1967).

V. Monoamine Oxidase Inhibitors

The chemistry, biochemistry and clinical pharmacology of MAO-inhibitors has been expertly reviewed by Pletscher et al. (1960), Biel et al. (1964) and Zirkle and Kaiser (1964).

The nearly accidental discovery of the antidepressant effect of iproniazid (Loomer et al., 1957), the first potent *in vivo* MAO-inhibitor (Zeller and Barsky, 1952), generated an unexpected interest in agents of this type. It was hoped that MAO-inhibitors would not only find therapeutic usefulness in psychoses but would also point to a solution of the etiology of mental disorders, principally because of their ability to prevent the metabolic breakdown of endogenous cerebral amines such as NE, 5-HT and dopamine. It was also suggestive to link the antidepressant effect of these substances with their biochemical effects. Such an hypothesis was corroborated by the already well known fact that reserpine, in contrast to MAO-inhibitors, depletes the brain of amines and not infrequently causes depression. However, since the physiologic significance of brain amines is not yet known (see chapter III, section C, 1 a) the explanation of the antidepressant effect of MAO-inhibitors must remain hypothetical, although evidence points to a causal relationship between antidepressant effect and enzyme inhibition (see Pletscher et al., 1960).

In spite of the fact that, at present, MAO-inhibitors have been largely replaced by the tricyclic compounds in the pharmaco-therapy of depression, a more detailed discussion of the pharmacology of the MAO-inhibitors seems to be justified, since they have played an important role in the development of the current hypotheses on the biochemistry of mental disorders (see above).

A. The Physiologic Significance of Monoamine Oxidase

The biochemistry and physiology of MAO has been extensively descussed by Blaschko (1952) and later by Davison (1958) and Pletscher et al. (1960).

MAO (synonyms: amine oxidase, tyraminase and adrenaline-oxidase) attacks a series of primary and secondary alkyl- and aralkyl-amines. By splitting off one molecule of ammonium, the corresponding carbonyl is formed:

$$R-CH_2-NH_3 + \tfrac{1}{2} O_2 \rightarrow R-CHO + NH_4 +$$

However, it has been demonstrated that during this oxidative deamination one molecule of H_2O_2 is formed which is split into H_2O and oxygen by utilizing unpurified, catalase-containing MAO preparations. The complete reaction is therefore as follows:

$$R-CH_2-NH\overset{+}{3} + O_2 + H_2O \xrightarrow{MAO} R-CHO + NH\overset{+}{4} + H_2O_2$$
$$\downarrow \text{catalase}$$
$$H_2O + \tfrac{1}{2} O_2$$

According to Zeller and Fouts (1963), the primary reaction product is not the aldehyde but the corresponding imino derivative R—C—CH = NH which is hydrolyzed to R—CHO and NH_3. The aldehyde is generally further oxidized to the carbonic acid (tyramine→p-hydroxyphenylacetic acid; dopamine→3,4-dihydroxyphenyl acetic acid; epinephrine and norepinephrine → 3,4-dihydroxymandelic acid) or rarely to the alcohol. The latter pathway seems to be important in rat and man since a substantial portion of epinephrine and norepinephrine is excreted as 3-methoxy-4-hydroxyphenyl glycol in the urine of these species (Axelrod et al., 1959; Goldstein et al., 1960; Kopin and Axelrod, 1960; Labrosse and Hertting, 1960). The MAO-activity in various organs of mammals changes from species to species. In most animals the highest MAO-activity is found in liver, kidney and nervous system (particularly autonomic ganglia). In contrast, little activity is found in heart, pancreas and thyroid gland. Amine oxidases occur in plasma of many mammals, but their significance is not clear (see Blaschko, 1962; Buffoni and Blaschko, 1964; Buffoni, 1966).

In cells, MAO is predominantly but not exclusively bound to mitochondria. The regional distribution of MAO in brain is not as specific as that of some of its substrates such as NE, dopamine or 5-HT (Birkhäuser, 1940; Bogdanski et al., 1957).

Among the many potential MAO-substrates, epinephrine, NE, dopamine and also tyramine, 5-HT, tryptamine and octopamine are of physiological interest. Of these endogenous substrates, dopamine and tyramine are metabolized at the fastest rate and epinephrine and NE at the slowest rate. 5-HT is metabolized at a rate somewhere between these two extreme groups (compare Pletscher et al., 1960).

The physiological significance of MAO is by no means clear, though it is certain that the enzyme plays a role in the degradation and detoxification of many monoamines formed in various organs. In particular, the significance of MAO in the inactivation of the above mentioned physiologically important amines has been discussed. Recent experiments, summarized by Kopin (1964), indicate that the NE which is more firmly bound to storage granules in nerves and which is released either by physiological turnover or by reserpine mainly undergoes oxidative deamination. The less firmly bound and exogenous NE and the NE which is released by nerve stimulation or tyramine is preferentially O-methylated by the enzyme O-methyl-transferase (see Axelrod, 1959). Thereby the corresponding methyl ethers of catecholamines are formed, e. g., 3-methoxy-norepinephrine (normetanephrine), 3-methoxy-epinephrine (metanephrine), 3-methoxy-dopamine (3-

methoxytyramine). These intermediate products are deaminated by MAO to aldehydes, which are further metabolized to either alcohols or the corresponding acids, e. g., 3-methoxy-4-hydroxy-mandelic acid (vanillyl-mandelic acid), 3-methoxy-4-hydroxyphenyl acetic acid (homovanillic acid) or 3-methoxy-4-hydroxyphenylglycol. The significance of MAO for the metabolism of the physiologically occurring amines is also stressed by the fact that inhibitors of this enzyme markedly increase amine concentration in brain and other organs of many species. Under physiological conditions a small portion of intracellular amines is present in unbound form in the cell plasma and is in equilibrium with the firmly bound intragranular amine portion. Since the unbound amine portion is constantly metabolized by MAO, it is conceivable that an important function of this enzyme is the maintenance of a diffusion gradient in the direction of unbound amines. This intracellular regulatory mechanism is necessary to maintain a constant amine concentration in the cell in spite of a continuous synthesis and storage of amines. According to this hypothesis, which is supported by many investigators (compare, e. g., Brodie and Beavan, 1963), MAO also regulates the amine concentration of intracellular stores. Inhibition of MAO causes an increase of the unbound amine and consequently leads to a diminution of the diffusion gradient for intragranular amines which results in a higher concentration of amines stored within the cell.

In this connection, it has to be mentioned that other pathways of degradation and inactivation exist, e. g., conjugation with sulfuric and glucuronic acids, oxidation to adrenochrome or N-acetylation.

B. Classification of MAO-inhibitors and their Structure-activity Relationship

One has to distinguish between those substances which inhibit MAO preferentially or exclusively *in vitro* and those which are also (or solely) active *in vivo*. The concentration necessary for inhibitors only effective *in vitro* is generally high (10^{-2} to 10^{-4} mol.). Among this type of inhibitors are d-amphetamine, ephedrine, cocaine, procaine, pentamidine, p-toluolcholine ester, diphenhydramine and many others (see Pletscher et al., 1960). The inhibition by these chemically heterogeneous compounds is either competitive and reversible or, less often, noncompetitive and irreversible. None of these agents has achieved practical significance as a MAO-inhibitor. It seems to be established that the pharmacologic effects of amphetamine and cocaine are not related to their MAO inhibitory property as has previously been assumed.

To the strong *in vivo* inhibitors of MAO belongs a group of chemically diverse agents, such as the hydrazines (incl. hydrazones, hydrazids, semicarbazides and thiosemicarbazides), harmala alkaloids, substituted indole alkylamines, propargylamines, cyclopropylamines and aminopyrazines. Most of these agents markedly inhibit MAO *in vitro* as well. However, significant qualitative differences exist: The inhibition by hydrazines, propargylamines and cyclopropylamines occurs only after prior incubation with tissue extract, that is after enzymatic transformation to active metabolites (also compare this chapter, section D), whereas the other substances do not require incubation in order to become active.

For practical purposes the inhibitors can be classified as long-lasting (mostly irreversible inhibition) and short-lasting (reversible inhibition). Long-lasting MAO-inhibitors are particularly hydrazine derivatives, aminopyrazines (2-methyl-3-piperidinopyrazine), cyclopropylamines (tranylcypromine), propargylamines (pargyline). Short-lasting inhibitors are harmala-alkaloids and substituted indolalkylamines (α-ethyltryptamine) (for literature reference, see Zirkle and Kaiser, 1964). Practically all these agents are competitive inhibitors.

Structure-activity relationships cannot be discussed here in great detail, and the reader is referred to extensive publications dealing with this problem (Pletscher et al., 1960; Biel et al., 1964; Zirkle and Kaiser, 1964).

1. Hydrazine Derivatives

The hydrazine type of MAO-inhibitor requires the following general chemical structure (Zeller et al., 1955): R—NH—NH—R'. R and R' can be varied extensively as long as one of the substituents contains an alkyl or substituted alkyl group. This makes it understandable why hydrazine itself, as well as phenylhydrazines or heterocyclic hydrazines (e. g., pyridylhydrazines), are inactive as inhibitors. The optimal effectiveness for alkyl- and aralkylhydrazine (NH_2—NH—R) requires a 2—4 carbon chain. To this group belong substances which are chemically closely related to the natural amine substrates of MAO, such as β-phenyl-isopropylhydrazine ($R = CH[CH_3]-CH_2—C_6H_5$) and benzylhydrazine ($R = CH_2-C_6H_5$). These highly active inhibitors have a great affinity for the enzyme.

Strong MAO-inhibitors are also found in the group of hydrazides (acylated hydrazines), e. g. iproniazid (1-isonicotinyl-2-isopropyl hydrazine). The general structure of this type of inhibitor is: R—CO—NR'—NH—R". It should be noted, however, that there are also compounds in this group which are completely devoid of MAO-inhibiting properties. The alkyl- and aralkylhydrazine moiety is responsible for the inhibitory effect whereas the acid function influences mostly the organ distribution and hydrolysis. Other highly effective hydrazides are the following: nialamide (2-[2-benzyl carb-amyl ethyl]-hydrazid isonicotinic acid) and isocarboxazide[1-benzyl-2-(5-methyl-3-iso-oxazolyl-carbonyl)hydrazine]. Acylation of both nitrogens in the hydrazine molecule abolishes the MAO-inhibitory effect.

2. Harmala-alkaloids

Among the harmala-alkaloids, harmine and harmaline are the most active inhibitors. Hydrogenation (= tetrahydroharmane and tetra-hydroharmaline) markedly reduces activity. Introduction of hydroxy groups into the aromatic ring (harmol, harmalol) also abolishes the inhibitory effect (Udenfriend et al., 1958; Pletscher et al., 1959 a).

3. Indolylalkylamines

Alkyl substitution at the α-carbon of tryptamine, which itself is a substrate for MAO, yields potent MAO-inhibitors, e. g., α-methyl- and α-ethyl-tryptamine (Vane, 1959; Greig et al., 1959; Gey and Pletscher, 1962 b). N-methylation of tryptamine (e. g., N,N-di-methyltryptamine) also produces MAO-inhibitors (Barlow, 1961). Additional substitution of α-alkyltryptamines on the indole ring considerably diminishes activity. Contrary to the original assumption of Wooley and Edelman (1958), 1-benzyl-5-methoxy-2-methyl-tryptamine (BAS) does not inhibit MAO in vivo (Tedeschi et al., 1959 b).

4. Propargylamines

N-methyl-N-2-propynylbenzylamine (pargyline) is a very potent MAO-inhibitor in vitro and in vivo. The N-methyl substitution is important for this effect since analogs with ethyl, phenyl and carbethoxy groups are less active. Equally important is the 2-pro-pynyl substituent. N-propyl and N-allyl derivatives are inactive. Substitution on the benzyl ring may increase or decrease activity but does not fundamentally alter the inhibitory effect (compare Zirkle and Kaiser, 1964).

5. Cyclopropylamine

2-Phenylcyclopropylamine (tranylcypromine) is 2—3 times more active in the ± trans-form than in the cis-form. On the other hand, the cis-2-phenoxycyclopropylamine has a greater inhibitory effect than the trans-isomer. Important for MAO-inhibition is the cyclopropane ring and substitutions in the 2-position. Substitution on the benzyl ring or N-atom may induce minor changes in activity without being critical for the MAO-inhibitory action.

6. Aminopyrazine

2-Methyl-3-piperidinopyrazine is an active inhibitor *in vivo* (Gylys et al., 1963; Dubnick et al., 1963), but its *in vitro* activity is weak. Essential for MAO-inhibiting properties is the presence of an alkyl group (e. g., 2-methyl) in the vicinity of the tertiary nitrogen (of the piperidinyl group). Absence or different location of this group leads to loss of activity. The piperidinyl group on the other hand, can be replaced by pyrrolidinyl, homopiperidinyl or morpholinyl without loss in activity (compare Zirkle and Kaiser, 1964).

7. Structural Similarities to Endogenous Amines

In order to understand the biochemical and pharmacological effects of many MAO-inhibitors, it is important to recognize their structural similarity to many amine substrates of this enzyme. Changing an amine, which could serve as a potential substrate, into the corresponding hydrazine often leads to enhancement of MAO-inhibition. This is exemplified in the case of amphetamine and phenylisopropylhydrazine. Zeller et al. (1955) and Fouts (1963) have defined the MAO-inhibiting hydrazines as "pseudoamines" which react with the same active center of the MAO-molecule as the true amine substrates. The structural analogy of MAO-inhibitors is also evident in the group of substituted tryptamines and cyclopropylamines.

Because of the chemical similarity between many MAO-inhibitors and sympathomimetic amine substrates, it is not suprising that many inhibitors possess sympathomimetic or sympatholytic properties. Such effects may be either direct or may involve displacement at receptor sites and release of catecholamines from their cellular binding sites. For example, β-phenylisopropyl hydrazine, tranylcypromine and α-alkyltryptamines possess amphetamine-like central activity (Eltherington and Horita, 1960; Vane et al., 1961; Van der Schoot et al.,

1962). Under certain conditions iproniazid induces receptor blockade (Griesemer et al., 1955) and releases NE from storage sites as does tranylcypromine (Goldberg and Shideman, 1962). Therefore, sympathomimetic or sympathicolytic effects (or side-effects) have to be expected during treatment with MAO-inhibitors. These side-effects may also markedly influence the effects due to enzyme inhibition in that the release of endogenous amines may partially or completely antagonize the accumulation of amines induced by MAO-inhibitors in tissues.

Pletscher et al. (1960) have extensively reported on the influence of MAO-inhibitors on enzyme systems other than MAO (diamine oxidase and other types of amine oxidases; amino acid decarboxylases; choline oxidase; succinic acid oxidase; DPN-ase, and many others).

C. Biochemical and Pharmacologic Effects of MAO-inhibitors

In consideration of above mentioned statements (B, 7) the following actions can be attributed to MAO-inhibitors: 1. They increase the concentration of endogenous and exogenous monoamines in many organs, particularly in brain. 2. They enhance the pharmacological effects of endogenous and exogenous monoamines. 3. Under certain conditions they antagonize the biochemical and pharmacological effects of reserpine in that they inhibit reserpine-induced amine release and prevent the central effects of reserpine and its analogs. 4. In man, most MAO-inhibitors have a more or less pronounced anti-depressant effect. 5. In addition, MAO-inhibitors have remarkable peripheral effects such as hypotension and may improve angina pectoris among others. It is tempting to speculate that all effects listed under points one to four are due to inhibition of MAO. In many instances it is possible to establish a satisfactory correlation between MAO-inhibition and effect. However, at present it is still uncertain if there is a relationship between MAO-inhibition and anti-depressant activity, although considerable evidence favors such a connection.

1. Biochemical Effects of MAO-inhibition

a) Effects on Monoamine Metabolism

The influence of MAO-inhibitors on the monoamine content varies from species to species and from organ to organ. Udenfriend et al. (1957) first demonstrated an increase of 5-HT in rat and rabbit brain after a single injection of iproniazid (see also Pletscher, 1956 a).

NE (Pletscher, 1957 a) and dopamine (Holzer and Hornykiewicz, 1959) concentration in brain of several species is similarly affected by iproniazid as well as by harmane derivatives, although the increase of these amines is never as pronounced as that of 5-HT. An increase in the concentration of normetanephrine and 3-methoxytyramine is found in mice as a consequence of MAO-inhibition (Carlsson et al., 1960). In contrast, cats and dogs do not respond to iproniazid with an increase in cerebral NE (Vogt, 1959; Spector et al., 1960 b). The catecholamine content of peripheral organs is increased by MAO-inhibitors in several species, e. g., in the heart of rat, guinea pig and dog (Muscholl, 1959; Pletscher, 1958; Crout et al., 1961). It remains, however, unchanged in the heart of rabbits and mice (Brodie et al., 1959 b; Leroy and Schaepdryver, 1961) and most tissues of cats (von Euler and Hellner-Bjorkman, 1955). Iproniazid increases the 5-HT concentration of the following organs: ileum of guinea pigs and rabbits, but not of rats (Pletscher, 1956 b), isolated perfused superior cervical ganglion of the cat (Gertner et al., 1957), blood of rabbit and blood platelets of man (Pletscher and Bernstein, 1958; Shore et al., 1958). Most MAO-inhibitors have effects similar to those of iproniazid. Some, however, such as tranylcypromine, pheniprazine and phenelzine, release NE from the heart (Lee et al., 1961; Goldberg and Shideman, 1962), whereas tranylcypromine liberates NE also from brain (Carlsson et al., 1960) (see also this chapter, section B, 7).

The onset of MAO-inhibition is generally very slow with the exception of that produced by pheniprazine and pargyline (Everett and Wiegand, 1961). The maximal increase in monoamines generally is reached 6—8 hours after administration. The following MAO-inhibitors have a faster onset of action (approximately 1 hour): harmane derivatives (Udenfriend et al., 1958), tranylcypromine (Tedeschi et al., 1960), α-ethyltryptamine (Greig et al., 1961) and 2-methyl-3-piperidinopyrazine (Dubnick et al., 1963; Gylys et al., 1963). Because of the relatively rapid onset of action, the maximal increase of amines induced by these inhibitors is reached earlier. The duration of action varies. Thus, MAO-inhibition induced by hydrazines (and also pheniprazine) lasts for several days and is of longer duration than the increase in amines. Equally long lasting in their effect are pargyline and 2-methyl-3-piperidinopyrazine, whereas tranylcypromine's effect appears to be of somewhat shorter duration. Harmane derivatives and α-ethyltryptamine have transient effects of a few hours duration. Repeated administration of small ineffective doses of hydrazines will produce a cumulative effect due to the long duration of activity, resulting in a measurable increase in brain monoamines. This finding is of great importance when MAO-inhibitors are to be administered clinically. Gey and Pletscher (1961 c) have called attention to the important fact that MAO must be inhibited at least by 80% in order to achieve a significant increase in brain monoamine concentration.

Certain monoamines, normally completely metabolized, accumulate in tissues after administration of MAO-inhibitors. Thus tryptamine (Hess et al., 1959), octopamine (Kakimoto and Armstrong, 1962) and β-phenylethylamine (Nakajima et al., 1964) accumulate in various organs after administration of iproniazid or pheniprazine. Many effects of MAO-inhibitors could be due to accumulation of these monoamines (compare this chapter, section C, 2 b).

b) *Metabolism of Exogenous Monoamines and their Precursors after Administration of MAO-inhibitors*

Pretreatment with MAO-inhibitors increases the accumulation of exogenous monoamines or their precursors in tissues. Thus, after pretreatment with iproniazid injection of NE and 5-HT leads to an increase in the concentration of these substances in rat heart (Pletscher et al., 1960).

Since NE, dopamine and 5-HT do not penetrate the blood brain barrier in significant amounts, the amine concentration in the brain has been raised by administering the precursors L-DOPA and 5-HTP. Effective MAO-inhibitors significantly increase the precursor-induced enhancement of the content of 5-HT (Udenfriend et al., 1957; Pletscher et al., 1960), NE and dopamine (Carlsson et al., 1958; Carlsson, 1959; Vogt, 1959). In contrast, substances with weak inhibiting properties such as isoniazid, harmalol, p-tolylcholinether and cocaine are devoid of this effect (see Pletscher et al., 1960). Pretreatment with MAO-inhibitors also markedly enhances the increase of tryptamine, o- and m-tyramine from their respective precursors in brain of rats and guinea pigs (Mitoma et al., 1957; Hess et al., 1959).

c) *The Excretion of Endogenous and Exogenous Monoamines and their Metabolites after Administration of MAO-inhibitors*

After prolonged treatment with MAO-inhibitors, the excretory profile of *endogenous* monoamines and their metabolites changes due to the inhibition of the enzyme. Under these conditions, the excretion of catecholamines and 5-HT increases but that of their metabolites, 3-methoxy-4-hydroxymandelic acid, homovanillic acid and 5-hydroxyindoleacetic acid decreases. The effects of MAO-inhibitors on the excretion pattern of catecholamines and 5-HT are less dramatic (compare Sjoerdsma et al., 1959 a; Pletscher et al., 1960) than those on the excretion of other amines such as tryptamine, p-(and perhaps m-)tyramine (Sjoerdsma et al., 1959 a), β-(4-hydroxyphenyl)-α-methylaminoethanol (Pisano et al., 1961), octopamine (Kakimoto and Armstrong, 1962) and β-phenylethylamine (Oates et al., 1963). The differences in excretion of the various amines are most probably due to the fact that tryptamine, tyramine and phenylethylamine are mainly deaminated by MAO, while catecholamines and 5-HT can be inactivated by other pathways. The measurement of an increase in tryptamine excretion in man has been recommended as a reliable *in vivo* test for MAO-inhibition in peripheral organs (Sjoerdsma et al., 1959 b; Sjoerdsma et al., 1960).

The excretion of metabolites deriving from exogenous catecholamines and 5-HT in urine is influenced more markedly than the excretion of endogenous material. After pretreatment with MAO-inhibitors and subsequent administration of dopamine, NE and epinephrine, the urinary excretion of homovanillic acid, 3,4-dihydroxyphenylacetic acid, 3-methoxy-4-hydroxymandelic acid and 3,4-dihydroxymandelic acid is much more reduced than in non-pretreated controls, while the concentration of free, conjugated and o-methylated substances (metanephrine, normetanephrine, 3-methoxytyramine), as well as of N-acetylated metabolites, increases (Goldstein and Musacchio, 1963). Also, secretion of 5-hydroxyindoleacetic acid, which is normally formed from exogenous 5-HT, is reduced after pretreatment with MAO-inhibitors as compared to controls, resulting in an increased excretion of 5-HT-glucoronide in rats (but not in man!). (For extensive literature references cf. Pletscher et al., 1960).

MAO-inhibitors do not alter the turnover rate of 5-HT in mice (Udenfriend et al., 1957, 1958) and of NE in mice (Udenfriend et al., 1959) and man (Friend et al.) but do prolong the half-life of injected tyramine and tryptamine. This is probably due to the differing significance of MAO for the various amines.

d) Antagonism between MAO-inhibitors of Short and Long Duration

Pletscher and Besendorf (1959) have demonstrated that the rise of amine concentration in brain induced by the irreversible inhibitor iproniazid can be prevented by pretreatment of the animals with the short-lasting, reversible inhibitor harmaline. Other short-lasting inhibitors, such as harmine (Horita and McGrath, 1960) and methylene blue (Ehringer et al., 1961), are also *in vivo* antagonists. It is assumed that both types of inhibitors occupy the same receptor sites of the enzyme molecule so that the long-lasting inhibitor of the hydrazid-type is ineffective when the critical site is taken by the short-lasting inhibitor. Evidence for this interpretation is the finding that certain combinations of harmala-alkaloids with MAO-inhibitors of long duration not only prevent the rise in amine content of various tissues but also abolish the inhibitory effect on the enzyme. In sharp contrast is the result of Ehringer et al. (1961) that harmine does not protect MAO from the inhibiting effect of iproniazid, though the 5-HT and NE increase in brain is prevented. However, certain combinations of MAO-inhibitors such as harmaline-iproniazid (Spector et al., 1960 a) and harmine-pheniprazine (Horita and McGrath, 1960) appear to protect MAO from the effect of the irreversible inhibitors. These discrepancies find a partial explanation in the findings of Horita and Chinn (1964). These authors showed that harmaline's inhibitory effect is longer lasting than that of harmine, and on the other hand, pheniprazine remains in tissues in its active form for a considerably shorter time than iproniazid. While harmaline protects MAO from iproniazid by virtue of its longer lasting inhibitory effect, harmine is devoid of this effect. Harmine, however, protects MAO from pheniprazine because pheniprazine disappears from tissue more rapidly than iproniazid. Nevertheless, the question remains unsolved as to why these complicated inter-actions between short- and long-lasting MAO-inhibitors primarily affect the activity of the enzyme *per se*, while the increase in amines induced by long-lasting inhibitors is prevented to a similar extent by harmaline and harmine. It is possible that the increase in amine con-centration only occurs when MAO-inhibition is very marked or that other effects of MAO-inhibitors, such as permeability changes and increase of storage capacity, play a significant role (see this chapter section C, 1 f).

e) Antagonism between MAO-inhibitors and Reserpine

The antagonism between MAO-inhibitors and reserpine is one of the most interesting biochemical and pharmacologic problems in this field, though the mechanism of this interaction has not been fully elucidated. Brodie et al. (1956 a), Chessin et al. (1956, 1957), and Besendorf and Pletscher (1956) were the first to observe that animals which are pretreated with effective doses of an MAO-inhibitor do not respond to reserpine with sedation and decreased locomotor activity but exhibit signs of central excitation. In addition pretreatment with iproniazid prevents reserpine-induced depletion of cerebral catecholamines and 5-HT (Brodie et al., 1956 a; Pletscher, 1956 a, b; 1957 b). Other MAO-inhibitors have a similar effect (for literature reference, see Pletscher et al., 1960; Zirkle and Kaiser, 1964). Short-lasting inhibitors have to be administered at a shorter interval before reserpine than long-lasting inhibitors. An antagonism similar to that against reserpine also exists between MAO-inhibitors and benzoquinolizine derivatives (Pletscher et al., 1958). It is noteworthy that in the cat hypothalamus iproniazid pretreatment does not prevent NE depletion induced by reserpine (Vogt, 1959). This is of particular interest since, in contrast to other species, iproniazid does not increase brain NE concentration in the cat (vide this chapter, C 1, a).

Combination of MAO-inhibitors and reserpine has a similar effect in peripheral organs such as the heart, ileum and adrenal cortex. However, the peripheral antagonism is less marked than in the brain and is dependent on the species (Holz et al., 1957 a). The antagonism can also be demonstrated with histochemical techniques (Zbinden et al., 1957 b; Zbinden and Studer, 1958). The antagonistic effect between MAO-inhibitors and reserpine is partially reversible. If MAO-inhibitors are administered during the maximal effect of reserpine, cerebral monoamines often increase. The increase of 5-HT is particularly significant under these conditions, whereas the increase of NE is less marked. Short-lasting inhibitors cause only a transient increase of the diminished 5-HT content, and the concentration of 5-HT soon drops to values which would be expected by giving reserpine alone (Pletscher et al., 1960). This appears to be due to the long-lasting effect of reserpine.

f) Mechanism of the Biochemical Effects of MAO-inhibitors

It is attractive to explain the above described effects of MAO-inhibitors (a—d) and their interaction with reserpine (e) as consequences of inhibition of the enzymatic degradation of endogenous and, particularly, exogenous (c) amines. In consideration of the fact that the key function of MAO is probably the maintenance of a constant amine level in cells (see this chapter, section A), the following additional statements can be made: 1. MAO-inhibition leads to an accumulation of free amines which are not bound in cellular storage sites. The concentration gradient of amines between storage sites and extragranular sites, and the diffusion of amines are therefore diminished. It can be expected that the intragranular amine content rises until the normal concentration gradient is reached again. 2. The antagonism between MAO-inhibitors and reserpine can be interpreted by assuming that the amines liberated from their stores by reserpine are not metabolized when MAO is inhibited and cannot leave the cells or synaptic area. It is known that free amines cannot penetrate the lipoid cell membrane as easily as the corresponding non-ionized aldehydes (see Zeller and Fouts, 1963).

Attempts to support this hypothesis by demonstrating shifts in the intracellular distribution of brain amines after administration of MAO-inhibitors have yielded controversial results. Giarman and Schanberg (1958) have consistently found an increase in the free amine fraction of brain homogenates after treatment with MAO-inhibitors, with or without reserpine, a finding which could not be confirmed by Weil-Malherbe and Bone (1959), Green and Erickson (1960), and Green and Sawyer (1960).

Although most data concerning the influence of MAO-inhibitors on amine content of various organs are considered to be a consequence of enzyme inhibition, some recent experiments point to another explanation. Thus, the above mentioned finding that harmine inhibits the iproniazid-induced increase of amines in rat brain but not the long-lasting MAO-inhibition of iproniazid itself indicates that two different mechanisms may be operating (Ehringer et al., 1961). Pepeu et al. (1961) have shown that following complete MAO-inhibition in guinea pig atria by suitable doses of iproniazid or pheniprazine, iproniazid prevented the spontaneous decrease of endogenous catecholamines much more effectively than pheniprazine. Axelrod et al. (1961 a) have noted that pheniprazine, pargyline and harmaline block the spontaneous slow release as well as the reserpine-induced fast release of exogenous H^3-NE stored in the heart. Therefore, the authors express the view that the increase in amine concentration in response to MAO-inhibitors also involves inhibition of release mechanisms. On the other hand, Zeller and Fouts (1963) believe that the findings of Axelrod et al. (1961 a) permit another explanation not in conflict with the MAO-concept. A new aspect is introduced by the finding that MAO-inhibitors not only increase endogenous NE in tissues but also other amines, e. g., octopamine. Since octopamine, according to Kopin et al. (1964), can act as a "false transmitter", it is released together with NE in proportion to its relative concentration. This may at least partly explain the diminished release of NE after MAO-inhibition found by Axelrod et al. (1961 a).

A study by Dubnick et al. (1962) shows that the increase of brain amines by MAO-inhibitors does not solely depend on enzyme inhibition. A comparison between iproniazid and phenelzine indicates that after administration of both agents in doses which completely block MAO of the mouse brain *in vivo*, phenelzine induces a greater increase in 5-HT than iproniazid. Twenty-four hours later the 5-HT content is diminished by 50%, whereas MAO remains completely inhibited. A second injection of phenelzine again causes an increase in 5-HT. Consequently, it must be assumed that the phenelzine-induced increase in 5-HT is not exclusively due to MAO-inhibition. Gey et al. (1963) have recently again studied a large number of MAO-inhibitors comparing doses causing 100% rise of 5-HT in the rat brain and 50% inhibition of MAO. From this comparison, the authors conclude that many MAO-inhibitors such as tranylcypromine, pheniprazine and nialamide not only raise the amine content by MAO-inhibition but also by influencing cellular amine binding, either by an increase of the storage capacity or by inhibition of amine release.

2. Pharmacological Effects of MAO-inhibitors

a) Central Effects

In order to understand the pharmacological effects of MAO-inhibitors on cerebral functions, it is important to realize the marked differences with which various species respond to this type of agent. While an explanation for this difference is not always at hand, one may assume that the significance of MAO for the metabolism of various amines differs from species to species. Moreover, several side-effects (see this chapter, section B, 7) inherent in the structure of certain MAO-inhibitors such as sympathomimetic, sympatholytic or monoamine releasing properties may also markedly modifiy the over-all effect depending on the species.

α) *Effect on Locomotor Activity.* In most species MAO-inhibitors tend to increase spontaneous motor activity. This effect is often seen only after repeated treatment for several days (Brodie et al., 1959). In contrast, a single dose of iproniazid may even have a "sedative" effect (see e. g., Brodie et al., 1959 a).

Several findings make it likely that the locomotor hyperactivity caused by MAO-inhibitors is related more to an increase in NE than in 5-HT. In this connection, particularly the following two findings must be mentioned: 1. In cats iproniazid predominantly increases 5-HT with insignificant effects on NE. In this species iproniazid does not cause excitation but rather exerts a calming effect (Vogt, 1959). A similar effect has been described in dogs (Brodie et al., 1959 b). 2. Brodie et al. (1959 b) have observed that treatment of rabbits with iproniazid, phenylisopropylhydrazine or phenylisobutylhydrazine for several days leads to a more pronounced increase in brain NE than a corresponding single dose. After a single injection the behavior of the animals remains unaltered, but multiple treatment significantly increases spontaneous activity. After termination of treatment the hyperactivity gradually subsides parallel to the brain NE content, while the 5-HT concentration remains high. A relationship between hyperactivity and NE concentration is, however, not proven since nialamide has been reported to cause hyperactivity in cats without an increase in brain NE (Funderburk, et al., 1962).

β) Effect on Spontaneous and Learned Behavior. Brimblecombe and Green (1962) have found that the behavior of untrained rats in Hall's open field situation, is influenced by MAO-inhibitors in direct proportion to their inhibiting effect *in vivo.* The duration of the effect also parallels the enzyme inhibition. The conditioned avoidance response is generally diminished or blocked by MAO-inhibitors, whereas the escape response is unaffected (for literature see Pletscher et al., 1960). It is, however, not certain if this effect is related to enzyme inhibition or to an increase in cerebral amines, since the sympathomimetics, such as catecholamines and amphetamines, as well as catechol precursors, such as L-DOPA, often exert the opposite effect on conditioned and unconditioned reflexes. Moreover, the effect occurs within such a short time after injection of the MAO-inhibitor that a significant increase in amines could not have taken place.

On the other hand, Olds and Olds (1958) have observed that in rats in which electrical self-stimulation of various brain areas is attained by bar pressing, MAO-inhibitors have an effect similar to that of catecholamines.

γ) Influence on Electrical Activity of the Brain. The effect of MAO-inhibitors on the EEG has been summarized in several reviews (see Pletscher et al., 1960; Werner, 1962; Killam, 1962). Generally it is assumed that MAO-inhibitors do not significantly alter the EEG. In very large doses, iproniazid may elicit an arousal response in rabbits. According to Costa et al. (1960), pheniprazine and tranyl-cypromine desynchronize the cortical potentials. A similar effect has been described for methyl- and ethyltryptamine (Himwich, 1961; Matthews et al., 1961). All these MAO-inhibitors possess amphet-amine-like, central stimulant properties which are probably respon-sible for the EEG activation rather than the enzyme inhibition *per se* or the increase in cerebral amines. However, Costa et al. (1960) assume, on the basis of their experiments, that the EEG changes parallel an increase in brain 5-HT. On the other hand, Shimizu et al. (1964), who have confirmed the EEG-activation of pheniprazine, believe that an increase in catecholamines is important for this effect. Everett (1961), who has described an arousal response to pargyline in rabbits, also assumes that this effect is due to a rise in brain dopamine and NE. Funderburk et al. (1962) have made the interesting observa-tion that nialamide, iproniazid and carboxazid induce spindling and slow waves in cats with chronically implanted electrodes. Further-more, nialamide does not alter the threshold for the direct stimulation of the ascending reticular system and the stimulation of the hippo-campus; it does, however, diminish the hippocampal after-discharges.

The transcallosal response is not only diminished by NE and 5-HT, but also by MAO-inhibitors, e. g., iproniazid (Marazzi, 1957). The interpretation of these findings is, however, difficult, even though the observation was made on a relatively simple synaptic system (compare Werner, 1962).

δ) Influence on the Central Effects of Amines and their Precursors. Many amines cause, when injected, various pharmacological effects which are in part due to an action on the CNS. Thus, phenylethyl-amine, 5-HT and mescaline raise the rectal temperature in rabbits, while epinephrine is practically inactive in this respect. 5-HT and tryptamine prolong hexobarbital sleeping time in mice. Ortho- and m-tyrosine stimulate the adrenergic system, and i. v. injection of tryptamine causes convulsions. All these effects of exogenous amines are potentiated by MAO-inhibitors (literature reference, see Pletscher et al., 1960). It is probable that the potentiating effects are due to inhibition of metabolism, since all these amines are substrates of MAO.

However, not all of the above described effects can be central in nature, because some of these amines, e. g., 5-HT, enter the brain only to a very limited extent.

Aminoacids such as DOPA, 5-HTP, o- and m-tyrosine, which are the precursors of their corresponding amines (dopamine, 5-HT, o- and m-tyramine), pass the blood brain barrier easily. The pharmacologic effects of the precursors, such as motor hyperexcitability, tremors and convulsions, can be regarded as predominantly central in nature and probably are the consequence of accumulation in the CNS of the corresponding amines. These effects are also potentiated by MAO-inhibitors (for literature reference, see Pletscher et al., 1960).

In mice, small doses of DOPA *per se* causes piloerection without changes in behavior or locomotor activity. When pretreated with a MAO-inhibitor, the same doses of DOPA evoke aggressiveness and marked hyperexcitability. This effect has been utilized by Everett and Wiegand (1962) to develop a simple screening test for such substances.

ε) *Influence on the Central Effects of Reserpine and Reserpine-like Agents.* Nearly all central pharmacological effects of reserpine and reserpine-like agents (e. g., benzoquinolizine derivatives) are diminished or abolished by pretreatment with effective doses of MAO-inhibitors. Sometimes, even a "reversal effect" occurs. Thus reserpine, after pretreatment with iproniazid, does not cause sedation, hypo-kinesia, hypothermia or parasympathetic dominance (ptosis, miosis) but, on the contrary, it evokes central stimulation, piloerection, hyperthermia and mydriasis (Brodie et al., 1956; Besendorf and Pletscher, 1956). Iproniazid and other MAO-inhibitors also reverse the reserpine-induced lowering of the threshold for electroshock in rats (Prockop et al., 1959) and pentylenetetrazol in mice (Hertting, 1958). Similarly, pentylenetetrazol toxicity, which is enhanced by reserpine, is normalized by iproniazid. As already mentioned (see chapter III, section C, 1 d), reserpine depletes the brain of GABA, which may be causally linked to the epileptogenic effect of reserpine (Balzer et al., 1961 a). Both phenomena are prevented by pretreatment with iproniazid. Iproniazid also antagonizes the reserpine-induced attenuation of morphine analgesia (Schaumann, 1958; Sigg et al., 1958).

Also of interest is the manner in which iproniazid pretreatment alters the reserpine effects on the EEG. Reserpine *per se* enhances the excitability of the non-specific intralaminar thalamic projection system, whereas after pretreatment with iproniazid, a significant increase in the excitability of the ascending reticular formation occurs (Tissot and Monnier, 1958). According to Werner (1962), this may indicate that reserpine generally releases more 5-HT which, like exogenous 5-HTP, causes slow wave activity in the EEG; after pretreatment with iproniazid, the ratio of amines released by reserpine may be shifted in favor of catecholamines thus inducing an arousal response.

An important study on the antagonism between tetrabenazine and various MAO-inhibitors has been published by Heise and Boff (1962). After pretreatment with MAO-inhibitors a standard dose of tetrabenazine is less effective in diminishing the conditioned response of rats in the Sidman-avoidance procedure than in non-pretreated animals. Since the tetrabenazine effect only lasts for a few hours, its activity can be tested repeatedly in the same animal. The authors have shown that the antagonistic effect of iproniazid reaches a maximum after 4 hours and lasts for many days. Even after 30 days, residual activity has been uncovered. Similar findings have been made with isocarboxazid, whereas harmaline was effective only for the duration of 8 hours. Harmaline, even when given several times at 24 hour intervals, did not have a cumulative effect. In contrast, cumulation occurred with iproniazid even when administered in 72 hour intervals. The intensity and duration of the pharmacological effect paralleled the enzyme inhibiting activity.

The pharmacological antagonism between MAO-inhibitors and reserpine is well correlated with the already described biochemical antagonism (this chapter, section C, 1 e). Thus, iproniazid prevents the central behavioral and amine releasing effects of reserpine more effectively if it is administered 16 hours prior to reserpine. On the other hand, if iproniazid is injected after reserpine administration, the sedative effect is only antagonized if a significant rise in brain amines has already occurred (Pletscher, 1957 b). It should be noted, however, that MAO-inhibitors which possess central amphetamine-like properties, such as 2-phenyl-cyclopropylamine (tranylcypromine), exert a strong antagonistic effect to reserpine even if administered after reserpine. This type of central antagonism is not due to an influence on amine metabolism but must be regarded as the consequence of a direct central stimulant effect of these agents.

The reported findings strongly indicate that the antagonism between MAO-inhibitors and reserpine is due to the antagonistic action on brain monoamine metabolism. On the basis of the various biochemical results (see this chapter, section C, 1 e, f), it must be assumed that, after inhibition of MAO, reserpine causes an increase in the concentration of free amines. This would not only explain the attenuation of the reserpine effects but also the reserpine "reversal". Indirect evidence for this assumption has been obtained by Pletscher et al. (1960). Combined administration of DOPA and 5-HTP, from which, particularly after MAO-inhibition, dopamine and 5-HT is formed in brain, produced pharmacological effects similar to those induced by combined treatment with iproniazid and reserpine. The correlation between these physiological and pharmacological effects not only contributes to a better understanding of the mechanism of action of these substances but also calls attention to the potential physiological significance of amines in cerebral function. Therefore, the effects described in this paragraph provide the basis for most of the hypotheses on brain amines and brain function (see chapter III, section C, 1 a, α, β, γ).

ζ) *The Anticonvulsant Effect.* Convulsions elicited by supramaximal electroshock are inhibited by pretreatment with various MAO-inhibitors. This effect and the increase in brain monoamines appear to parallel each other (Prockop et al., 1959). A similar effect is observed in mice (Chow and Hendley, 1959). In contrast, pentylenetetrazole-induced seizures in mice do not seem to be influenced by pretreatment with MAO-inhibitors (Hertting, 1958; Everett et al., 1959). Everett et al. (1959), however, have not been able to confirm the protective effect of MAO-inhibitors on electroshock. Clinically, the MAO-inhibitors do not play any role as anticonvulsants.

η) *Other Central Effects.* Some MAO-inhibitors of the hydrazine-type have been claimed to possess analgesic properties. This is a weak effect, however, and not related to the increase in brain amines (see Pletscher et al., 1960; Emele et al., 1961).

Several MAO-inhibitors prolong the barbiturate sleeping time (literature reference, see Pletscher et al., 1960). This effect reaches its maximum soon after administration and does not parallel MAO-inhibition; it is due to inhibition of barbiturate metabolizing enzymes in the liver microsomes (Laroche and Brodie, 1960). On the other hand, it is possible that the report of Holtz et al. (1957 b) describing a shortening of hexobarbital and tribromoethanol narcosis by MAO-inhibitors is related to the inhibition of MAO and the subsequent rise in brain amine content, since this effect occurs after considerable latency and relates better to the temporal sequence of the biochemical events.

b) Peripheral Effects

Details regarding the manifold peripheral effects of MAO-inhibitors can be found in the review of Pletscher et al. (1960). The increasing significance of some MAO-inhibitors in the treatment of hypertension makes it necessary to discuss briefly the hypotensive effect and its mechanism. Numerous MAO-inhibitors (iproniazid, nialamide, pargyline, harmaline) transiently lower arterial blood pressure in several species. The rapid onset of action makes it unlikely that this effect is related to enzyme inhibition. In the literature, several other possible explanations are discussed: 1. Blockade of ganglionic transmission which has been observed in the isolated superior cervical ganglion *in situ* (Gertner, 1961) and in the intact animal (Goldberg and Da Costa, 1960). 2. Schmitt and Gonnard (1956) report that the blood pressure response to epinephrine and NE is diminished by MAO-inhibitors. However, other authors have found that the vasopressor and nictitating membrane response to these amines is unaltered or slightly enhanced (Balzer and Holtz, 1956). The adrenolytic effect may be due either to competitive displacement of catecholamines from receptors (Griesemer et al., 1955) or to diminished sensitivity of the vessels to amines because of their increased endogenous NE-content (Pletscher et al., 1960). (It must be noted that the effect of other amines such as tyramine, tryptamine, 5-HT is enhanced by MAO-inhibitors [Balzer and Holtz, 1956]). 3. Gessa et al. (1963) have recently made the interesting observation that MAO-inhibitors have a "bretylium-like" effect at the adrenergic nerve endings, which means that, like bretylium, they inhibit liberation of NE induced by physiological impulses. This property, which does not apear to be related to enzyme inhibition, offers a new and different explanation for the blood pressure lowering effect of MAO-inhibitors. 4. It has already been mentioned that in many tissues inhibition of MAO leads to accumulation of amines which are, under physiological conditions, completely metabolized by MAO. Kopin et al. (1964) have shown that octopamine formed from tyramine after administration of pheniprazine may act as a "false transmitter" in the specific noradrenergic stores of adrenergic nerve endings. According to these authors, stimulation of these nerves would release less NE than normally because of the shift of equilibrium between the two amines in favor of octopamine. Since the effect of the released "false" transmitter is generally smaller than that of NE, the net effect is a diminution of the response to physiological stimuli (see also Fischer et al., 1965 a). It is possible that this mechanism may play a role in the lowering of blood pressure in man after prolonged treatment with MAO-inhibitors; it does not, however, explain the almost immediate onset of hypotension. It has also been considered whether or not accumulation of octopamine in the heart plays a role in the beneficial effect of MAO-inhibitors in angina pectoris (Kakimoto and Armstrong, 1962). Experimental attemps to find an explanation for the anti-anginal action of MAO-inhibitors have not been very successful. The following factors have been considered important: analgesia, ganglionic blockade, increase in blood lactic acid (Gey and Pletscher, 1960), diminution of the hemo-dynamic response to physical exertion (Horowitz et al., 1961), psychic stimulation and reduction of oxygen consumption in heart muscle.

Other peripheral effects of MAO-inhibitors are: increase in coronary flow, protection against experimentally-induced (particu-larly reserpine) stomach ulcers, inhibition of intestinal motility (see Pletscher et al., 1960).

D. Fate of MAO-inhibitors in the Body

Relatively little is known about the fate of MAO-inhibitors in the body. Iproniazid is apparently decomposed mainly to isopropyl-hydrazine and isonicotinic acid. It is not known if nialamide undergoes similar changes. It is possible that the potent inhibitory effect of iproniazid *in vivo* is due to the intermediate product, isopropyl-hydrazine, which is a strong MAO-inhibitor itself. In favor of this view is the finding that *in vitro* iproniazid is only effective when preincubated with tissue extracts. Isocarboxazid is very rapidly metabolized in the organism, hippuric acid being one of the break-down products which appears in urine. However, it is not certain whether *in vivo* the benzyl rest is split off or the benzylhydrazine as is the case under *in vitro* conditions. Pargyline is excreted in urine to a great extent unaltered. After treatment with tranylcypromine, hip-puric acid appears in urine. The harmane derivatives, such as harmaline, split off the aromatic methoxy groups forming hydroxy derivatives which are less active as inhibitors (e. g., harmalol) (for literature see Pletscher et al., 1960; Biel et al., 1964; Zirkle and Kaiser, 1964).

E. Adverse Reactions and Dangers

Pletscher et al. (1960), Hollister (1964) and Wagensommer (1964) have reported on the side-effects which are to be expected during clinical application of MAO-inhibitors. Maling et al. (1962) have published on the effect of chronic administration of relatively large doses of various MAO-inhibitors in dogs and on the resulting pathologic-anatomical changes.

1. Suicide and Fatal Poisoning

Hollister (1964) mentions a successful suicide with 500 mg tranylcypromine in a 17 year old girl. Marked central stimulation accompanied by delirium, tremor, profuse perspiration, coma, shock, heart block and hyperthermia preceded death which occurred 8 hours after ingestion of the drug.

2. Central Nervous System

The central side-effects which occur during prolonged treatment with MAO-inhibitors are manifold. Because of the central nervous stimulation, sleeplessness and agitation are frequent. Retarded depression may suddenly change to agitated depression. Hypomanic, delirious and confusional states as well as exacerbation of psychotic symptoms in schizophrenics can be observed during treatment with MAO-inhibitors. Epileptic episodes occur very rarely. Occasionally, the extrapyramidal motor system is affected in that choreiform hyperkinesia, which is striatal in nature, can be seen. However, the fine tremor, which sometimes can be detected, is not to be mistaken for extrapyramidal tremor.

3. Autonomic Nervous System

During treatment with MAO-inhibitors disturbances of the autonomic system occur very frequently: hypotension, tachycardia, dryness of the oral mucosa, hyperhydrosis, hot flashes, micturition difficulties, diarrhea, constipation and impotence. Rarely are these side-effects so marked that therapy has to be terminated.

4. Jaundice

The occurrence of jaundice during chronic administration of MAO-inhibitors is always serious. This side-effect is relatively frequent in regard to iproniazid (1 : 4000). Newer agents appear to cause icterus less frequently. However, jaundice has also been noted after nialamide, phenelzine, pheniprazine, tranylcypromine and ethyltryptamine. There is no reason to assume that the liver-damaging effect is due to MAO-inhibition. It therefore seems theoretically feasible to develop MAO-inhibitors without hepatotoxic side-effects. The clinical and pathologic-anatomical manifestations are those of viral hepatitis with diffuse damage to the liver parenchyma, from local necrosis of individual liver cells to the acute yellow liver atrophy. Mortality is greater than that of a viral hepatitis. Patients with a history of liver damage or suffering from it should be treated with MAO-inhibitors only if absolutely necessary and with extreme caution. Iproniazid and ethyltryptamine have been withdrawn from the market partly because of their liver damaging effect.

5. Miscellaneous Side-effects

Blood dyscrasias (leucocytosis, and also leucopenia and anemia) are rare. Cases of atrophy of the optic nerve, resulting in loss of vision or red-green color blindness, has so far only been observed with pheniprazine which has also been withdrawn from the market. It is unlikely that these side-effects are the consequence of MAO-inhibition.

6. Incompatibility

The occurrence of incompatibility of MAO-inhibitors with various other substances is of great practical significance. In patients undergoing treatment with MAO-inhibitors, thymoleptics (such as imipramine and amitriptyline) and reserpine or tetrabenazine, may cause delirium, disorientation, agitation, hallucinations, tachycardia, profuse sweating, mydriasis, cyanosis, hyperthermia, cardiovascular collapse and/or convulsions. Such combinations have had occasionally a lethal outcome (see Harrer, 1961). Ingestion of various types of cheeses and also broad beans by patients receiving MAO-inhibitors may cause complications, particularly hypertensive crises, mainly accompanied by severe headaches which are often localized in the occipital region. This type of side-effect has been most often noted with tranylcypromine although other MAO-inhibitors have also been implicated. Muscholl (1965) and Sjöqvist (1965) have reviewed the pertinent literature. Asatoor et al. (1963) have presented evidence that tyramine, which is present in large quantities in some cheeses, accumulates in the organism after inhibition by MAO and provokes the side-effects. Broad beans have been found to contain considerable amounts of DOPA. Patients who have been treated with iproniazid may exhibit alcohol intolerance.

7. Physical Dependence and Withdrawal

There is at present no evidence indicating that chronic treatment with MAO-inhibitors induces physical dependence or that withdrawal symptoms appear after termination of treatment. Cessation of drug administration may, however, cause increased psychomotor excitability, oppressive dreams, depression, nausea and vomiting.

8. Danger of Suicide

In patients, particularly those with retarded depression, who are under treatment with MAO-inhibitors, the incidence of attempted suicide is increased. This is not to be considered a side-effect of MAO-inhibitors but rather the consequence of successful therapy—namely the change from retarded to agitated depression.

VI. Thymoleptics

This class of psychotherapeutic drugs encompasses agents which are clinically useful antidepressants of the non-MAO-inhibitor type. Of practical significance in this group are the following tricyclic agents: iminodibenzyls (imipramine and desmethylimipramine), iminostilbenes (opipramol), dibenzocycloheptadienes (amitriptyline and its desmethyl derivative), dibenzodiazepines (dibenzepine), dibenzocycloheptatrienes (protriptyline), dihydroanthrazene-derivatives (melitracene).

The chemistry, pharmacology and clinical application of tricyclic thymoleptics has been reviewed *in extenso* by Häfliger and Burckhardt (1964).

A. Peripheral Effects

All thymoleptics lower blood pressure, transiently dependent on the dose administered. They also enhance and prolong a variety of responses induced by endogenous release and exogenous administration of NE. This has been demonstrated in many organs and for many species including man (Sigg, 1959; Haefely et al., 1964; Cairncross, 1965; Schmitt and Schmitt, 1966 b; Fishbach et al., 1966; for further literature see Häfliger and Burckhardt, 1964). Large doses, however, tend to have an adrenolytic effect. The difference between thymoleptics and phenothiazines is in this respect only quantitative since a catecholamine potentiating effect can, under special circumstances, also be observed with low doses of phenothiazines (Martin et al., 1960). In isolated tissues, only adrenolytic effects are observed with tricyclic antidepressants. The NE-enhancing effects may be explained on the basis of interference with uptake and binding mechanisms by these agents. The thymoleptics block the inactivation of amines by inhibiting the uptake of NE through the cell membrane of peripheral tissues (Hertting et al., 1961; Axelrod et al., 1961 b; Carlsson and Waldeck, 1965). This effect is not specific for the tricyclic antidepressants in that phenothiazines, adrenergic neuron blockers, antihistamines and cocaine exert a similar action. In contrast to NE, epinephrine responses are altered only to a minor extent by thymoleptics, whereas the effects of indirectly acting amines such as tyramine and amphetamine are generally diminished (Vernier et al., 1962; Kaumann and Basso, 1966; Schmitt and Schmitt, 1966 b). Thymoleptics do not inhibit the uptake of catecholamines into storage granules but appear to inhibit solely the uptake from the extra-neuronal space into the terminal adrenergic nerve fibers (Carlsson and Waldeck, 1965). This would indicate that thymoleptics, in contrast to reserpine (see chapter III, section B, 4 b), have no influence on the synthesis of NE from dopamine taking place in the granules.

Imipramine, amitriptyline and their desmethyl-derivatives also enhance some peripheral effects of serotonin (Sigg et al., 1963). On the other hand, many other 5-HT actions are diminished especially after administration of large doses. Thus the rat paw edema, gastric ulcer and the increased capillary permeability induced by 5-HT are reduced by tricyclic antidepressants (Domenjoz and Theobald, 1959; Mörsdorf and Bode, 1959; Theobald et al., 1964). The uptake of 5-HT into blood platelets is inhibited (Stacey, 1961), but this effect is not specific in that chlorpromazine and cocaine have a similar effect.

Thymoleptic agents possess a weak cholinolytic activity *in vitro* in the order of magnitude of that of the phenothiazines (Domenjoz and Theobald, 1959). However, *in vivo* the cholinolytic effects as evidenced by the antagonism of the hypotensive response to acetylcholine and vagal stimulation, as well as to pilocarpine-induced salivation, seem to be somewhat more pronounced (Theobald et al., 1965).

The substantial peripheral antihistaminic properties of tricyclic antidepressants *in vitro* (Theobald et al., 1964) and *in vivo* (Metysova et al., 1963; Theobald et al., 1964) led to the belief that central antihistaminergic properties might contribute to the clinical effectiveness of these agents. This viewpoint has been reinforced by the fact that several antihistamines also potentiate the responses to NE and inhibit catecholamine uptake (Isaac and Goth, 1965; Sigg and Hill, 1966).

However, clinically demonstrated antidepressant activity among thymoleptics seems to be inversely correlated to their antihistaminic potency.

B. Central Effects

1. Interaction with Central Autonomic Mechanisms

The interference of tricyclic antidepressants with peripheral adrenergic mechanisms, although not specific, led to the assumption that these agents also interfere with central adrenergic events which may be the basis for their clinical effectiveness (Sigg, 1959). Investigations of pharmacological interactions between antidepressants and central adrenergic agents (methylphenidate; cocaine; amphetamine; precursors of dopamine and norepinephrine; releasers of amines, e. g., tetrabenazine and reserpine; blockers of amine metabolism) have indeed provided considerable support for the biogenic amine theory of depression.

Many effects of central stimulants (e. g., amphetamine, methylphenidate and LSD) are enhanced by imipramine, desipramine and amitriptyline: for instance, motor hyperactivity in rodents (Halliwell et al., 1964), conditioned avoidance behavior (Carlton, 1961; Scheckel and Boff, 1964), increased rate of responding for rewarding hypothalamic stimulation (Stein and Seifter, 1961), hyperthermia (Jori and Garattini, 1965), methamphetamine-enhancement of evoked cortical potentials in rabbits (Plotnikoff and Everett, 1965). However, interpretation involving central adrenergic mechanisms should consider the recent evidence that the amphetamine potentiating effects in response to tricyclic antidepressants are at least in part due to an inhibition of amphetamine metabolism in brain (Sulser et al., 1966; Consolo et al., 1967). Hyperpyretic responses and stimulated behavior induced by DOPA in mice pretreated with a MAO-inhibitor are also increased by tricyclic antidepressants (Sigg and Hill, 1966; Everett, 1967). MAO-inhibitors combined with imipramine lead to fighting in mice (Sabelli et al., 1961) and to EEG arousal in dogs (Himwich and Peterson, 1961). Such interactions are of clinical importance because combinations of MAO-inhibitors with tricyclic antidepressants may result in serious CNS side effects (see this chapter, section D, 6).

A principal difference between phenothiazine-derivates and thymoleptics is the fact that the latter prevent the central depressant effects of reserpine and reserpine-like compounds. Reserpine and tetrabenazine have served as the foremost models in the laboratory to simulate a depressive state. It has been shown that the various symptoms induced by these two depressant agents can be prevented or antagonized by thymoleptics in many species: ptosis (Halliwell et al., 1964; Schmitt and Schmitt, 1966 a; Metyš and Metysova, 1967), hypothermia (Garattini et al., 1962; Votova et al., 1965), motor hypoactivity (Pöldinger, 1963; Sigg et al., 1965; Jori et al., 1966), prolongation of pentobarbital sleeping time in mice (Sulser et al., 1960). There is convincing evidence that adrenergic mechanisms are involved in the antagonism of reserpine or tetrabenazine by tricyclic antidepressants. Thymoleptics no longer antagonize reserpine effects after pretreatment with α-methyl-meta-tyrosine (a NE depleting agent) (Scheckel and Boff, 1964; Sulser et al., 1964). Furthermore, the hyperactivity induced by desipramine in the reserpinized animal can be blocked by centrally acting adrenolytic agents (Matussek et al., 1964). The mechanism of the interaction of thymoleptics with reserpine is rather complex. The tricyclic antidepressants do not prevent amine-depletion induced by reserpine in brain (Garattini et al., 1962; Pletscher and Gey, 1962). This indicates that these agents do not interfere with the loss of norepinephrine storage capacity in intraneuronal sites induced by reserpine. It has been shown that desipramine decreases the rate of norepinephrine disappearance caused by reserpine (Manara et al., 1966). This effect could be due to an increased rate of synthesis of norepinephrine coupled with impairment of reuptake through the cell membrane, thereby delaying depletion of norepinephrine (Manara et al., 1966; Neff and Costa, 1967). More direct evidence of an effect of tricyclic antidepressants on central adrenergic mechanisms has been provided by studies which indicate that the uptake of tritiated norepinephrine injected into the ventricals of rats is inhibited by certain thymoleptics (Glowinski and Axelrod, 1964). Of interest is the finding that the inhibition of uptake is most marked in the medulla oblongata, cerebellum and hypothalamus with minor or no change in the striatum, midbrain, hippocampus and cortex (Glowinski et al., 1966). Clinically inactive agents seem not to affect central norepinephrine uptake (Glowinski and Axelrod, 1964). This finding has been confirmed by histochemical fluorescence methods which reveal that imipramine-like agents inhibit the uptake of norepinephrine into central catecholamine fibers (Hamberger and Masuoka, 1965). An increased normetanephrine concentration after intracisternal injection of tritiated norepinephrine in rats is found after pretreatment with imipramine and its desmethylated derivatives (Schanberg et al., 1967). In this connection it is noteworthy that the excretion of normetanephrine increases during the recovery of depressed patients treated with imipramine (Schildkraut et al., 1965). In contrast, the uptake of intraventricularly injected 5-HT into 5-HT neurons of reserpine-nialamide pretreated rats is not blocked by desimipramine, given in doses which inhibit norepinephrine-uptake (Fuxe and Ungerstedt, 1967). While there is considerably less information available on the interference of antidepressant agents with central 5-HT, it is believed that serotonin plays a lesser role than catecholamines in the mechanism of action of antidepressant agents. This viewpoint is also based on indirect observations such as the weak reserpine antagonism of 5-HTP as compared to that of DOPA.

There is also no convincing evidence that the central cholinolytic action plays a significant role in the mechanism of action of antidepressant agents. A central cholinolytic effect has been assumed to be of importance because of the findings that EEG arousal evoked by eserine is diminshed (Bradley and Key, 1959; Benesova et al., 1964) and that tremorine-induced tremors are reduced by antidepressants (Rathbun and Slater, 1963; Theobald et al., 1964; Loew and Taeschler, 1965). Moreover, reserpine produces a parasympathico-mimetic syndrome, and its toxicity is enhanced by anticholine-sterase inhibitors and cholinergic drugs (Liebmann and Matthies, 1964). However, it was later demonstrated that the tremorine-antagonism by antidepressant agents is due to an inhibitory effect on the metabolism of tremorine to oxotremorine (Hammer and Sjö-qvist, 1967). Oxotremorine tremor is either unaltered or prolonged by antidepressants (Sjöqvist and Gillette, 1965; Meyts and Metysova, 1967). Moreover, atropine is only a weak antagonist to the central effects of reserpine (Askew, 1963). Other investigators also have failed to find a correlation between antireserpine and central cholinolytic action (Lapin, 1967; Metys and Metysova, 1967). Imipramine and amitriptyline do not antagonize the arecoline-induced tremor (Masak et al., 1965).

In conclusion, all the findings are so far compatible with the hypothesis that increased availability of norepinephrine at critical central sites may be the most important mechanism through which the antidepressant effect is achieved.

2. Effect on Behavior

In general, tricyclic antidepressant agents possess weak phenothiazine-like properties in animals. Therefore, very high doses of antidepressants are required to impair locomotor activity and somatic reflexes. Exploratory behavior of rodents placed in a Y-maze is not affected by imipramine (Marriott and Spencer, 1965). Experiments involving operant techniques also indicate that tricyclic antidepressants do not cause significant avoidance failures except in very high doses (Cook and Kelleher, 1962; Morpurgo, 1965; Owen and Rathbun, 1966).

3. Electrophysiologic Studies

Numerous studies indicate that the thymoleptics behave like weak phenothiazines in that they slow the frequency of the EEG and reduce the arousal reaction to various sensory stimuli (Sigg, 1959; Monnier and Krupp, 1959; Arrigo et al., 1962; Himwich et al., 1964). Although many electrophysiological data reported are confusing because of different species, time schedules and dosages used, most investigators have found an effect of thymoleptics on the rhinencephalon. Thus, imipramine and amitriptyline were found to shorten after-discharges in the amygdala (Mercier et al., 1963). Locally evoked amygdaloid potentials are diminished while at the same time evoked potentials in the mesencephalic reticular formation are increased (Guerrero-Figueroa and Gallant, 1967). The septal potential evoked by stimulation of the dorsal hippocampus is also markedly enhanced by amitriptyline, imipramine and their desmethyl analogs (Schmitt, 1967). Furthermore, in cats with permanently implanted electrodes it was found that imipramine not only enhances arousal discharges in the olfactory bulb to novel stimuli but also enhances reticular arousal by electrical stimulation (Rubio-Chevannier, 1961). These findings are of interest in connection with the behavioral response of killing by selected rats, a response which is dependent on intact amygdala and is inhibited by thymoleptics in doses well below those affecting motor equilibrium (Horovitz et al., 1965). Small doses of imipramine lower the threshold of the rage response to hypothalamic stimulation in cats (Penaloza-Rojas et al., 1961).

4. Other Central Effects

Tricyclic antidepressants lower body temperature in several species but do so to a considerably lesser extent than the phenothiazines (Sigg, 1959; Herr et al., 1961; Theobald et al., 1965). The anti-depressants lack any antiemetic effect against apomorphine and do not offer significant protection against electroshock, strychnine and penta-methylenetetrazol seizures (Theobald et al., 1965). Interaction with other CNS active agents varies greatly with species. In rodents either hexobarbital, pentobarbital, thiopental and ethanol sleeping times are slightly prolonged but to a considerably lesser extent than by neuroleptic agents (Domenjoz and Theobald, 1959; Herr et al., 1961; Frommel et al., 1962). In contrast, barbital and chloralhydrate hypnosis is not prolonged in dogs (Kato et al., 1963).

C. Metabolic Fate

The metabolism of amitriptyline and imipramine occurs in the liver and is effected by the microsomal enzyme system requiring $NADPH_2$ and O_2 (Dingell et al., 1964). Imipramine is metabolized by demethylation and hydroxylation with the subsequent formation of glucuronides (Herrmann et al., 1959; Herrmann, 1963). A comprehensive summary of some 16 possible pathways of imipramine metabolism has been recently published (Bickel and Baggiolini, 1966). Not only has desmethylated imipramine been isolated and identified in brain (Gillette et al., 1961) but it has also been shown that desipramine accumulates in tissues after administration of imipramine (Dingell et al., 1964). Desipramine seems to be somewhat more potent in certain pharmacological procedures but does not have a more rapid onset of action. The major metabolites of amitriptyline are also products of desmethylation and hydroxylation (Hucker, 1962). However, in contrast to imipramine and desmethyl-imipramine hydroxylation of amitriptyline occurs at the ethylene bridge. C^{14}-labelled amitriptyline and imipramine are rapidly concentrated in brain. Relatively high concentrations are also found in tissues where most side-effects occur, e. g., salivary and lachrymal glands, and gastrointestinal tract (Cassano and Hansson, 1966).

D. Adverse Reactions

Side-effects and complications, while relatively common with thymoleptic agents, are less threatening than those observed with MAO-inhibitors. Hollister (1964) and Wagensommer (1964) have reviewed side-effects and dangers in the use of thymoleptics.

1. Suicide and Poisoning

Successful suicides have been reported after ingestion of amitriptyline and imipramine. In most instances, large amounts up to several grams of the substance have been ingested. However, in the case of a child, imipramine in a dose of only 350 mg has caused death (Hollister, 1964). After large doses of imipramine, coma, clonic convulsions, shock, respiratory depression, fever and dysrhythmias are observed. Amitriptyline generally causes coma, tachycardia and hypothermia.

2. Central Nervous System

Therapeutic treatment with thymoleptics may cause side-effects similar to those seen after MAO-inhibitors, such as restlessness, insomnia, hypomania and delirious states. Thymoleptics, not infrequently, also produce toxic psychotic states seen very rarely during neuroleptic treatment. Rarely do extrapyramidal symptoms occur, although occasionally tremors (particularly of the tongue and hands) and choreiform hyperkinesias are noted. EEG changes have been recorded and epileptic seizures have occurred in predisposed patients.

3. Peripheral Side-effects

Peripheral side-effects of thymoleptics are frequent and manifold. A moderate hypotension with tiredness, lassitude, dizziness and blurred vision is most often observed. Occasionally imipramine induces thromboses (leg, pelvis) and emboli, which are probably related to a disturbance in vascular reactivity. A direct connection between thymoleptic therapy and the occurrence of myocardial infarction is not established though stenocardic complaints are sometimes voiced by cardiac patients receiving this treatment. Therapeutic doses of thymoleptics may also induce arrhythmias and ECG changes such as flattening of the T-wave and prolongation of the PQ-interval. Tachycardias are equally frequent. Of practical significance are those side-effects which are caused by the "atropine-like" effects of thymoleptics: aggravation of an existing glaucoma, urinary retention, micturition difficulties, dryness of the oral mucosa and constipation.

4. Allergic Dermatoses

Allergic dermatoses, photosensitization and pruritus may occur during imipramine treatment particularly in patients and medical attendants who are also hypersensitive to phenothiazines.

5. Agranulocytosis; Jaundice

The most serious but fortunately very rare complication of imipramine treatment is agranulocytosis which resembles, in its course, that induced by phenothiazines. Amitriptyline-induced agranulocytosis has also been reported but is even less frequent than that caused by imipramine. Jaundice, which occasionally erupts after imipramine, is less serious than the iproniazed jaundice. It is, like the phenothiazine jaundice, cholestatic in nature.

6. Incompatibilities

Patients under treatment with MAO-inhibitors may suffer very serious complications when concurrently given thymoleptics (see chapter V, section E, 6). Such combinations, particularly in large doses, may precipitate hypertensive crises and hyperthermia. If therapy with thymoleptics is necessary, it is indicated to delay treatment 10—14 days after termination of administration of MAO-inhibitors.

7. Withdrawal Symptoms

Sudden termination of thymoleptic therapy, particularly of imipramine treatment, may cause "withdrawal" symptoms such as restlessness, insomnia, nausea, vomiting and sweating.

VII. Chemical Structures, General Clinical Use and Daily Human Dose Range of the most Frequently Used Psychotherapeutic Drugs [1]

A. Antipsychotic (Neuroleptic) Agents

Clinical use: Phenothiazines are mainly used in treating conditions marked by excessive agitation as it occurs in some schizophrenic disorders, during the manic phase of manic-depressive psychosis, involutional and toxic (e. g. alcohol) psychoses. These agents may

---

[1] The daily dose ranges have been established by consulting the following references: *New drugs.* Ed. American Medical Association 1967. — *Physicians desk reference.* Medical Economics, Inc. 1968. — *Usdin, E., and D. H. Efron.:* Psychotropic drugs and related compounds. Public Health Service Publication No. 1589, U.S. Dept. of Health, Education and Welfare 1967. — *Pöldinger, W.:* Kompendium der Psychopharmakotherapie. Basel: F. Hoffmann-La Roche & Co. 1967. — *Goodman, L. S., and A. Gilman:* The pharmalogical basis of therapeutics. 3rd ed New York: The Macmillan Company 1966.

reduce hallucinations, delusions, panic, hostility and excitement of the psychotic patients. Because of their secondary pharmacological actions, some drugs of this class are in use in nonpsychiatric conditions as antiemetics, analgesics and adjuncts to general anesthesia. The thioxanthene derivatives, butyrophenones and reserpine essentially have the same clinical indications as the phenothiazines. The butyrophenones are claimed to be particularly useful for the treatment of the syndrome of Gilles de la Tourette.

1. Phenothiazine Derivatives

promethazine

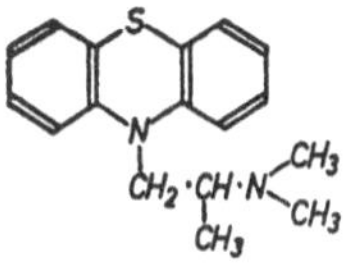

10-(2-dimethylaminopropyl)-phenothiazine
Dose: 12.5—50 mg (no antipsychotic activity)

promazine

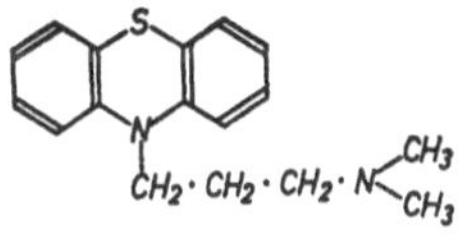

10-(3-dimethylaminopropyl)-phenothiazine
Dose: 75—200 mg, up to 1000 mg in hospitalized
patients

chlorpromazine

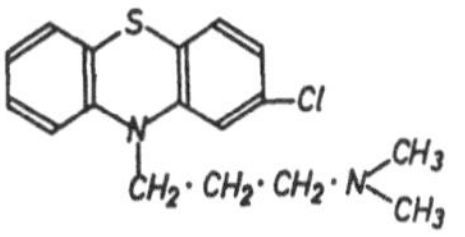

10-(3-dimethylaminopropyl)-2-chloropheno-
thiazine
Dose: 30—400 mg, up to 2000 mg in hospitalized
patients

methopromazine

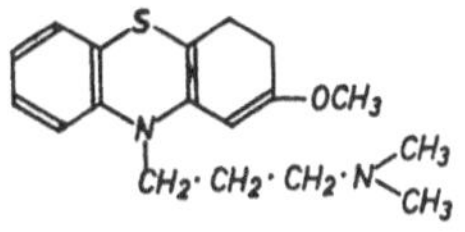

10-(3-dimethylaminopropyl)-2-methoxy-
phenothiazine
Dose: 30—1500 mg

acepromazine

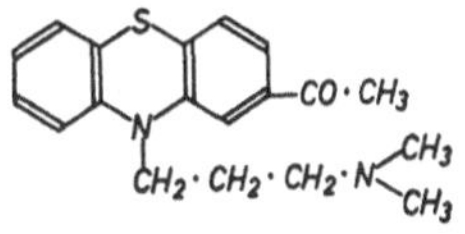

10-(3-dimethylaminopropyl)-2-acetyl-
phenothiazine
Dose: 60—90 mg in severe cases up to 200 mg

trifluopromazine

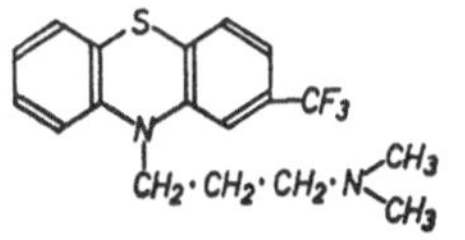

10-(3-dimethylaminopropyl)-2-trifluomethyl-
phenothiazine
Dose: 50—200 mg, up to 300 mg in severe cases

trimeprazine

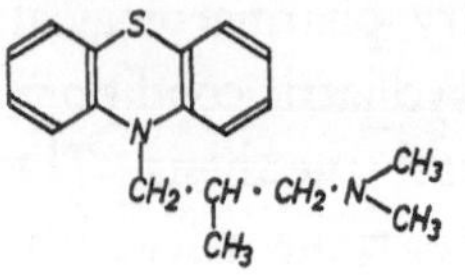

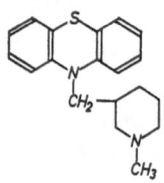

10-(3-dimethylamino-2-methylpropyl)-
phenothiazine
Dose: 2.5—10 mg

methotrimeprazine

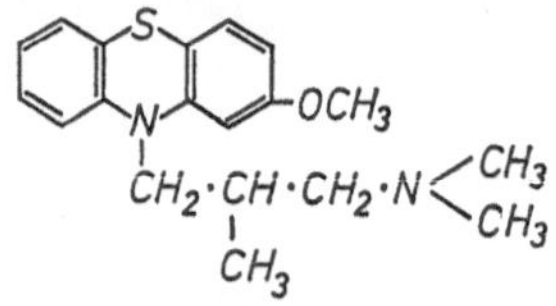

10-(3-dimethylamino-2-methylpropyl)-
2-methoxyphenothiazine
Dose: 25—1000 mg

b) Piperidylalkyl-phenothiazine Derivatives

mepazine

10-(1-methyl-3-piperidylmethyl-
phenothiazine
Dose: 75—200 mg, up to 600 mg in hospitalized
patients

thioridazine

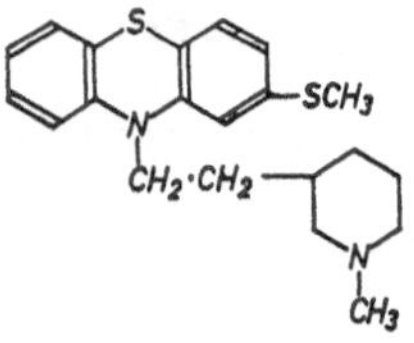

10-[2-(1-methyl-2-piperidyl)-ethyl]-2-methyl-
mercaptophenothiazine
Dose: 50—400 mg, up to 1600 mg in hospitalized
patients

c) Piperazinylalkyl-phenothiazine Derivatives

perazine

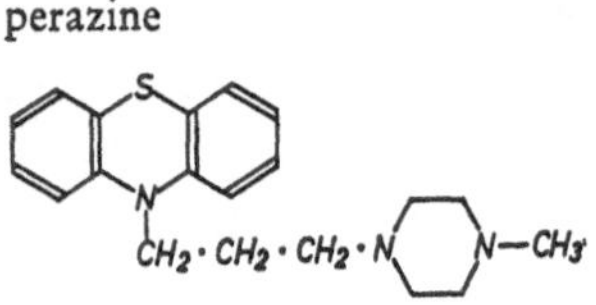

10-[3-(4-methyl-1-piperazinyl)-propyl]-
phenothiazine
Dose: 50—150 mg

prochlorperazine

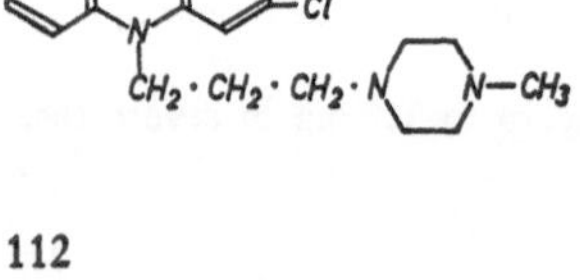

10-[3-(4-methylpiperazinyl)-propyl]-
2-chlorphenothiazine
Dose: 10—60 mg, up to 200 mg in hospitalized
patients

112

trifluoperazine

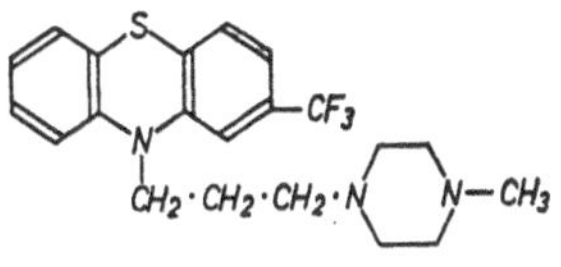

10-[3-(4-methyl-1-piperazinyl)-propyl]-2-trifluoromethylphenothiazine
Dose: 4—10 mg, up to 30 mg in hospitalized patients

perphenazine

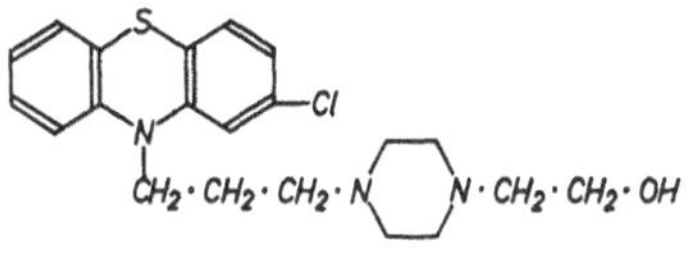

10-[3-(4-{2-hydroxyethylpiperazi-nyl)-propyl]-2-chlorophenothiazine
Dose: 8—24 mg, up to 64 mg in hospitalized patients

fluphenazine

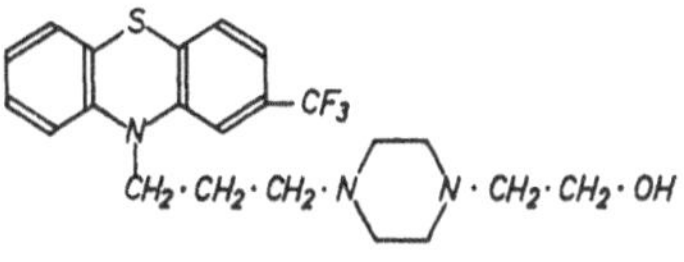

10-[3-(4-hydroxyethylpiperatinyl)-propyl]-2-fluoromethylphenothiazine
Dose: 1—3 mg, up to 20 mg in hospitalized patients

thiopropazate

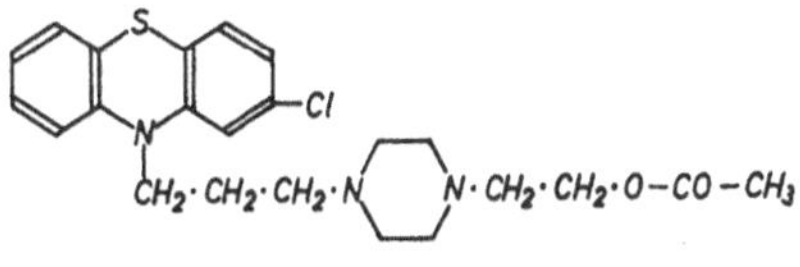

{3-[1-(2-acetoxyethyl]-4-piper-azinyl]-propyl}-2-chlorpheno-thiazine
Dose: 10—30 mg, up to 150 mg in hospitalized patients

2. Thioxanthene Derivatives

chlorprothixene

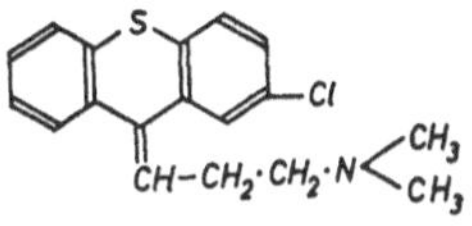

2-Chloro-9-(3-dimethylaminopropylidene)-thioxanthene
Dose: 45—200 mg

3. Butyrophenone

haloperidol

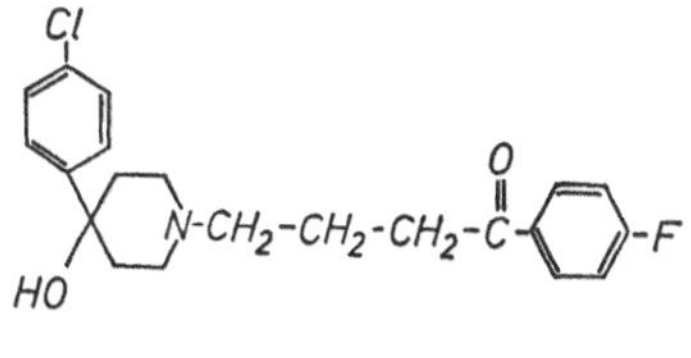

p-Fluoro-4-[4-hydroxy-4-(p-chlorophenyl)-piperidino]-butyrophenone
Dose: 0.5—9 mg

4. Reserpine and Reserpine-like Agents

reserpine

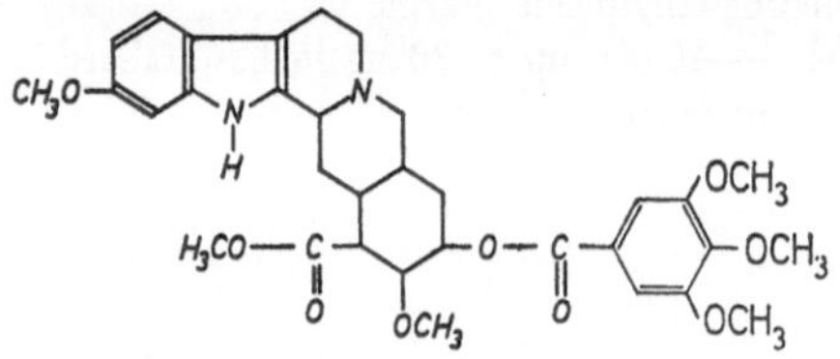

3,4,5-trimethoxybenzoyl-
methylreserpate
Dose: 0.1—1 mg

deserpidine

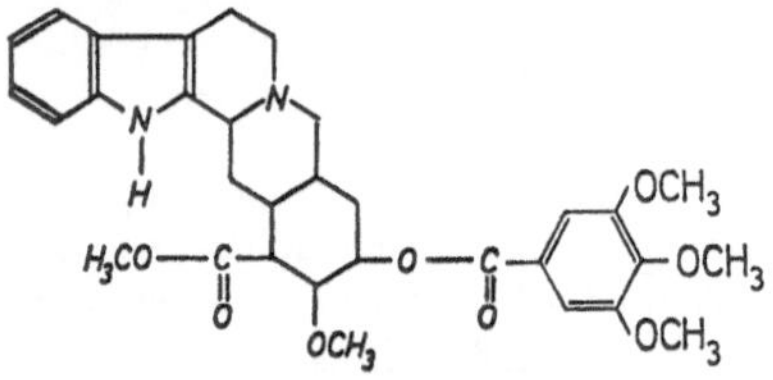

11-desmethoxyreserpine
Dose: 0.1—2 mg

syrosingopine

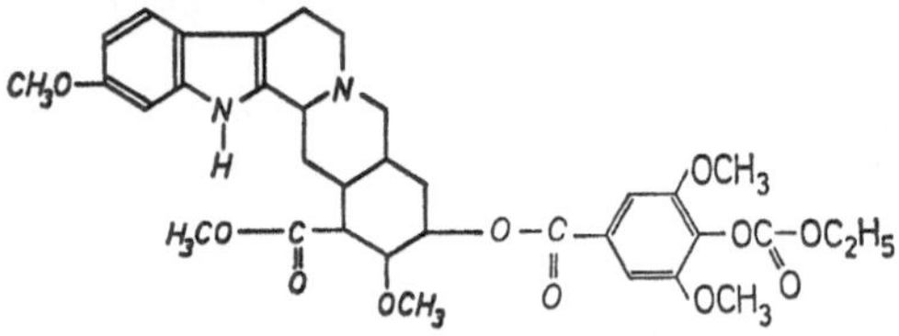

carbethoxysyringoylmethyl-
reserpate
Dose: 0.5—3 mg (used as antihypertensive agent only)

rescinnamine

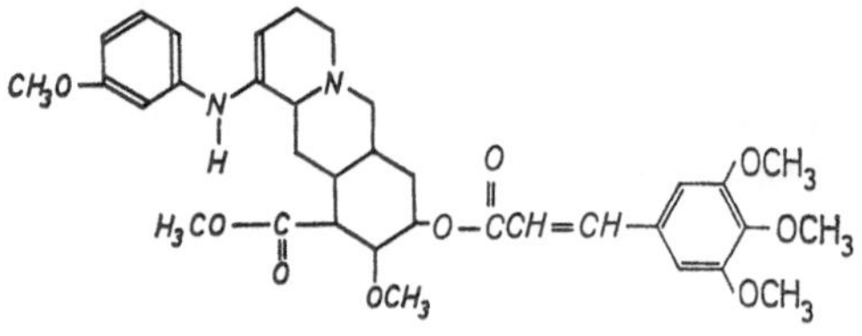

3,4,5-trimethoxycinnamoyl-
methylreserpate
Dose: 0.25—2 mg

tetrabenazine

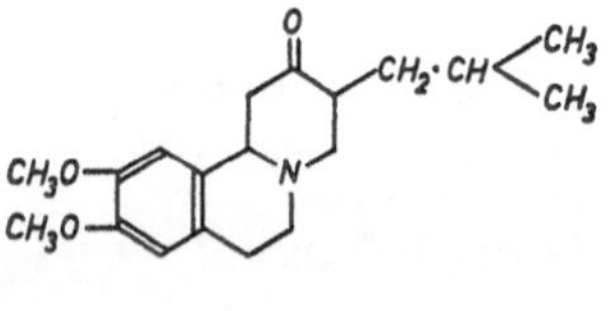

3-isobutyl-1,2,3,4,6,7-hexa-
hydro-11bH-benzo(a)quinoli-
zine-2-one
Dose: 25—200 mg

114

B. Antianxiety Agents (Minor Tranquilizers)

Clinical use: The minor tranquilizers are effective in the treatment of psychoneurotic and psychosomatic manifestations. They suppress anxiety, tension and help control excessive stress reactions. While they are not effective in controlling the disturbed psychotic patients, some of the more potent agents of this type may be helpful in the treatment of acute agitation in schizophrenics, toxic psychoses and during withdrawal from alcohol.

1. Propanediol—carbamates

meprobamate

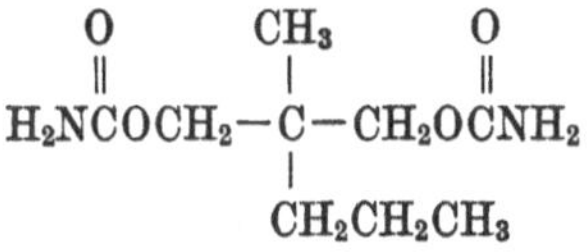

O
CH₃
O
H₂NCOCH₂—C—CH₂OCNH₂
CH₂CH₂CH₃

dicarbamate of 2-methyl-2-propyl-1,3-propanediol
Dose: up to 1600 mg

2. Benzodiazepines

chlordiazepoxide

NHCH3
N=C
CH2
Cl
C=N
O
C6H5

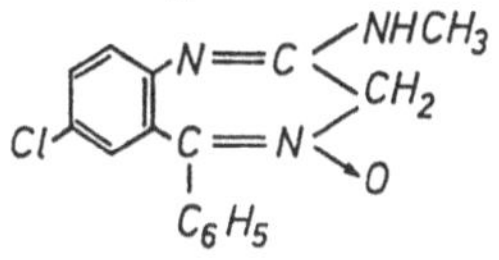

7-Chloro-2-methylamino-5-phenyl-3H-1,4-benzodiazepine-4-oxide-hydrochloride
Dose: 15—40 mg, up to 100 mg in severe cases

diazepam

CH3
N—CO
CH2
Cl
C=N
C6H5

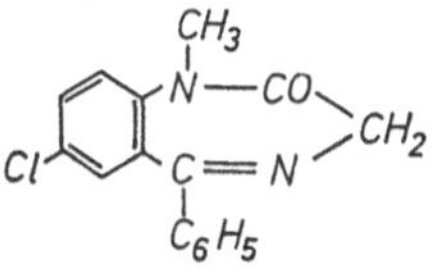

7-Chloro-1-methyl-5-phenyl-3H-1,4-benzodiazepin-2(1H)-one
Dose: 4—15 mg, up to 40 mg in severe cases

C. Antidepressants

Clinical use: This class of drugs, encompassing the MAO-inhibitors and tricyclic compounds are useful in the treatment of depression, particularly the endogenous type. They are also used alone or in conjunction with phenothiazines in the treatment of the depressive phase of certain types of schizophrenia.

1. MAO-inhibitors

iproniazid

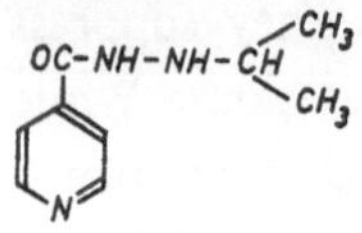

1-isonicotinoyl-2-isopropylhydrazine
Dose: 50—150 mg

isocarboxazid

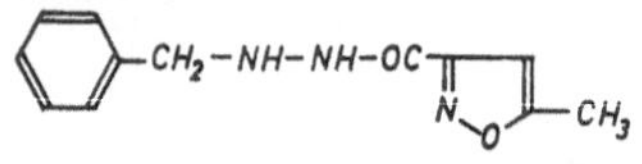

1-benzyl-2-(5-methyl-3-isoxazolylcarbonyl)-
hydrazine
Dose: 10—30 mg

nialamide

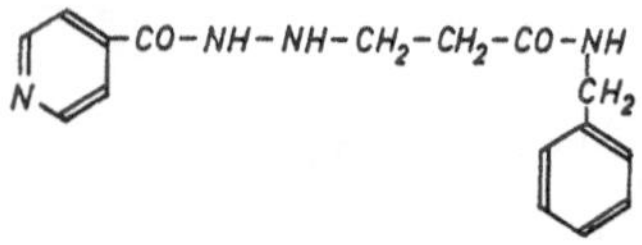

N-isonicotinoyl-N'-(β-N-benzylcarbox-
amidoethyl)-hydrazine
Dose: 25—150 mg

pheniprazine

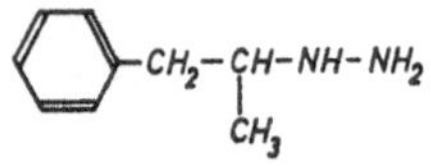

α-methyl-β-phenylethylhydrazine
Dose: 3—12 mg

phenelzine

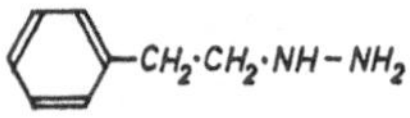

β-phenylethylhydrazine
Dose: 15—75 mg

tranylcypromine

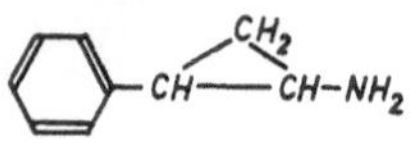

2-phenylcyclopropylamine
Dose: 20—40 mg

etryptamine

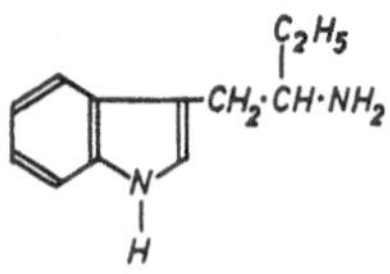

3-(2-Aminobutyl)-indole
Dose: 15—90 mg

pargyline

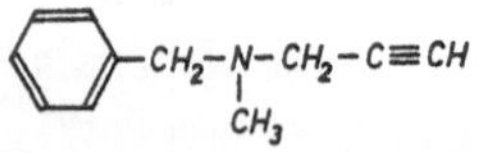

N-methyl-N-propargylbenzylamine
Dose: 25—150 mg (as antihypertensive)

2. Iminodibenzyls and Related Tricyclic Compounds

imipramine

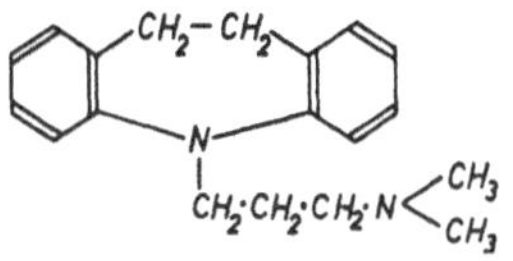

5-(3-dimethylaminopropyl)-10,11-dihydro-5H-dibenz[b,f]-azepine
Dose: 75—300 mg

trimepramine

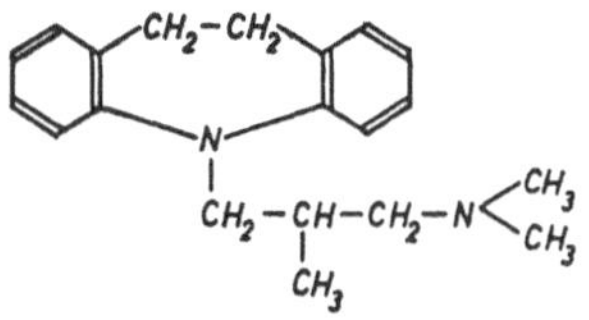

5-(3-dimethylamino-β-methyl-propyl)-10,11-dihydro-5H-dibenz-[b,f]-azepine
Dose: 75—300 mg

desipramine

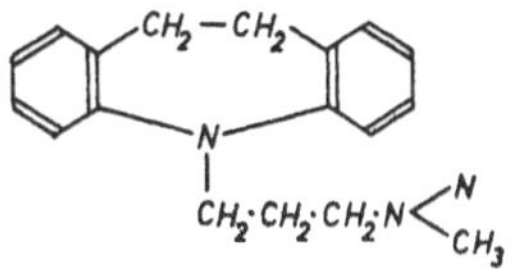

5-(3-methylaminopropyl)-10,11-dihydro-5H-dibenz-[b,f]-azepine
Dose: 75—200 mg

opipramol

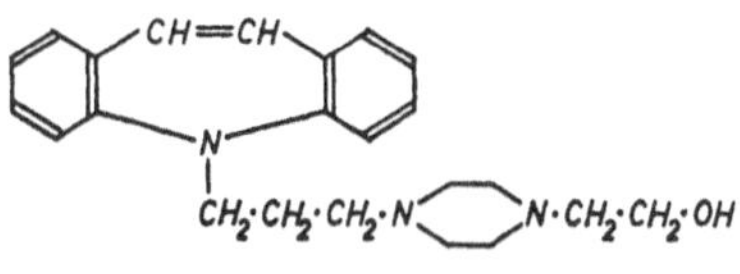

5-{γ-[4-(β-hydroxy-ethyl)piperazino]-propyl}-5H-dibenz-[b,f]-azepine
Dose: 25—300 mg

amitriptyline

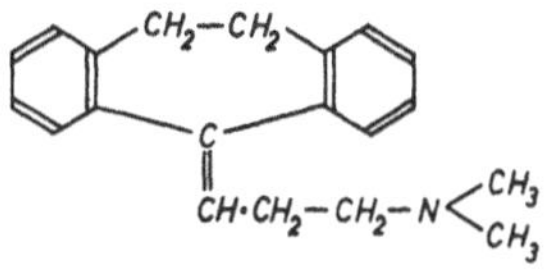

5-(3-dimethylaminopropylidene)-5H-dibenzo[a,d][1,4]-cycloheptadiene
Dose: 20—300 mg

nortriptyline

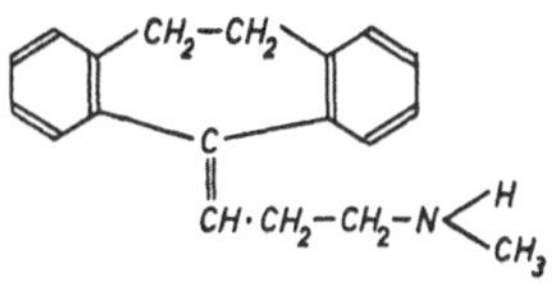

5-(3-methylaminopropylidene)-5H-dibenzo[a,d][1,4]-cycloheptadiene
Dose: 20—100 mg

Abbreviations

ACTH	=	adrenocorticotropic hormones of the anterior lobe of hypophysis
ADP	=	adenosinediphosphate
AMP	=	adenosinemonophosphate
ATP	=	adenosinetriphosphate
CPZ	=	chlorpromazine
L-DOPA	=	L-dihydroxyphenylalanine
Dopamine	=	3-hydroxytyramine = 3,4-dihydroxyphenylethylamine
ECG	=	electrocardiogram
EEG	=	electroencephalogram
FAD	=	flavinadenindinucleotide
GABA	=	γ-aminobutyric acid
5-HT	=	5-hydroxytryptamine serotonin
5-HTP	=	5-hydroxytryptophane
LSD	=	lysergic acid diethylamide
MAO	=	monoamineoxidase
NE	=	norepinephrine
Octopamine	=	4-hydroxyphenylethanolamine = β-hydroxytryramine
CNS	=	central nervous system

Bibliography

Abood, L. G., and K. L. Romanchek: *The chemical constitution and biochemical effects of psychotherapeutic and structurally related agents.* Ann. N. Y. Acad. Sci. 66, 812—825 (1957).

Adey, W. R., and C. W. Dunlop: *Amygdaloid and peripheral influences on caudate and pallidal units in the cat and effects of chlorpromazine.* Exp. Neurol. 2, 348—363 (1960).

Agranoff, B. W., R. M. Bradley, and J. Axelrod: *Determination and physiologic disposition of meprobamate.* Proc. Soc. exp. Biol. Med. 96, 261—264 (1957).

Aigner, A., O. Hornykiewicz, H.-T. Lisch, and A. Springer: *Beeinflussung der Gehirn-Katecholamine, der Spontanaktivität und der L-DOPA-Hyperaktivität durch Diäthyldithiocarbamat.* Med. Pharmacol. Exp. 7, 576—585 (1967).

Alexander, L., and S. R. Horner: *The effect of drugs on the conditional psychogalvanic reflex in man.* J. Neuropsychiat. 2, 246—261 (1961).

Amin, A. H., T. B. B. Crawford, and J. H. Gaddum: *The distribution of substance P and 5-hydroxytryptamine in the central nervous system of the dog.* J. Physiol. 126, 596—618 (1954).

Andén, N. E., A. Carlsson, and B. Waldeck: *Reserpine-resistant uptake mechanisms of noradrenaline in tissues.* Life Sci. 2, 889—894 (1963 a).

—, B. E. Roos, and B. Werdinius: *3,4-Dihydroxyphenylacetic acid in rabbit corpus striatum normally and after reserpine treatment.* Life Sci. 2, 319—325 (1963 b).

—, T. Magnusson, and B. Waldeck: *Correlation between noradrenaline uptake and adrenergic nerve function after reserpine treatment.* Life Sci. 3, 19—25 (1964 a).

—, B. E. Roos, and B. Werdinius: *Effects of chlorpromazine, haloperidol and reserpine on the levels of phenolic acids in rabbit corpus striatum.* Life Sci. 3, 149—158 (1964 b).

—, A. Carlsson, A. Dahlstrom, K. Fuxe, N. A. Hillarp, and K. Larsson: *Demonstration and mapping out of nigro-neostriatal dopamine neurons.* Life Sci. 3, 523 to 530 (1964 c).

Anderson, E. G., and D. D. Bonnycastle: *A study of the central depressant action of pentobarbital, phenobarbital and diethylether in relationship to increases in brain 5-hydroxytryptamine.* J. Pharmacol. exp. Ther. 130, 138—143 (1960).

Arellano, Z. A. P., and V. R. Jeri: *Scalp and basal EEG during the effect of reserpine.* Arch. Neurol. Psychiat. 75, 525—533 (1956).

Arnold, O. H.: *Personal communication.*

Arrigo, A., V. Cosi, F. Savoldi et M. Tartara: *Modificazioni indotte dall'amitriptilina sull'attivita elettrica cerebrale spontanea ed evocata del coniglio non anestetizzato.* Boll. Soc. ital. Biol. sper. 38, 621—624 (1962).

—, G. Jann, and P. Tonali: *Some aspects of the action of Valium and of Librium on the elecrical activity of the rabbit brain.* Arch. int. Pharmacodyn. 154, 364—373 (1965).

Arrigoni-Martelli, E., et M. Kramer: *Studio farmacologico di un nuovo derivato fenotiazinico: la perfenazina.* Arch. int. Pharmacodyn. 119, 311—333 (1959).

Asatoor, A. M., A. J. Levi, and M. D. Milne: *Tranylcypromine and cheese.* Lancet, 2, 733—734 (1963).

Askew, B. M.: *A simple screening procedure for imipramine-like antidepressant agents.* Life Sci. 2, 725—730 (1963).

Axelrod, J.: *Metabolism of epinephrine and other sympathomimetic amines.* Physiol. Rev. 39, 751—776 (1959).

—, I. J. Kopin, and J. D. Mann: *3-Methoxy-4-hydroxyphenylglycol sulfate, a new metabolite of epinephrine and norepinephrine.* Biochem. biophys. Acta. 36, 576—577 (1959).

—, G. Hertting, and R. W. Patrick: *Inhibition of H^3-norepinephrine release by monoamine oxidase inhibitors.* J. Pharmacol. exp. Ther. 134, 325—328 (1961 a).

—, C. G. Whitby, and G. Hertting: *Effect of psychotropic drugs on the uptake of H^3-norepinephrine by tissues.* Science 133, 383—384 (1961 b).

Ayd, F. J.: *A survey of drug-induced extrapyramidal reactions.* JAMA 175, 1054—1060 (1961).

Bain, J. A., and S. E. Mayer: *Biochemical mechanisms of drug action.* Ann. Rev. Pharmacol. 2, 37—66 (1962).

Baker, R. V.: *Observations on the localization of 5-hydroxytryptamine.* J. Physiol. 142, 563—570 (1958).

—, H. Blaschko, and G. V. R. Born: *The isolation from blood platelets of particles containing 5-hydroxytryptamine and adenosine triphosphate.* J. Physiol. 149, 55—56 (1959).

Balzer, H., u. P. Holtz: *Beeinflussung der Wirkung biogener Amine durch Hemmung der Aminoxydase.* Naunyn-Schmiedeberg Arch. exp. Path. 227, 547—558 (1956).

— — u. D. Palm: *Reserpin und α-Amino-buttersäuregehalt des Gehirns.* Experientia 17, 38—40 (1961 a).

— — — *Reserpin und Glykogengehalt der Organe.* Experientia 17, 304—305 (1961 b).

Barbeau, A., G. F. Murphy, and T. L. Sourkes: *Excretion of dopamine in disease of basal ganglia.* Science 133, 1706—1707 (1961).

—, T. L. Sourkes et G. F. Murphy: *Les catecholamines dans la maladie de Parkinson.* In: Monoamines et systeme nerveux central. Ed. J. de Ajuriaguerra. Paris: Masson; Geneve: Georg, pp. 247—262 (1962).

Barlow, R. B.: *Effects on amine oxidase of substances which antagonize 5-hydroxytryptamine more than tryptamine on the rat fundus strip.* Brit. J. Pharmacol. 16, 153—162 (1961).

Barraclough, C. A.: *Blockade of the release of pituitary gonadotrophin by reserpine.* Fed. Proc. 14, 9—10 (1955).

—, and C. H. Sawyer: *Induction of pseudopregnancy in the rat by reserpine and chlorpromazine.* Endocrinology 65, 563—571 (1959).

Bartlet, A. L.: *The 5-hydroxytryptamine content of mouse brain and whole mice after treatment with some drugs affecting the central nervous system.* Brit. J. Pharmacol. 15, 140—146 (1960).

Bastian, J. W.: *Classification of CNS drugs by a mouse screening battery.* Arch. int. Pharmacodyn. 133, 347—364 (1961).

Behn, W., M. Frahm u. E. Fretwurst: *Über den diaplacentaren Übergang von Phenothiazin-Derivaten.* Klin. Wschr. 34, 872 (1956).

Bein, H. J., F. Gross, J. Tripod u. R. Meier: *Experimentelle Untersuchungen über „Serpasil" (Reserpin), ein neues, sehr wirksames Rauwolfiaalkaloid mit neuartiger zentraler Wirkung.* Schweiz. med. Wschr. 83, 1007—1012 (1953).

Bein, H. J.: *Significance of selected central mechanisms for the analysis of the action of reserpine.* Ann. N. Y. Acad. Sci. 61, 4—16 (1955).

— *The pharmacology of rauwolfia.* Pharmacol. Rev. 8, 435—483 (1956).

Bejrablaya, D., J. H. Burn, and J. M. Walker: *The action of sympathomimetic amines on heart rate in relation to the effect of reserpine.* Brit. J. Pharmacol. 13, 461—466 (1958).

Benditt, E. P.: Diskussionsbemerkung in: G. P. Lewis: *5-Hydroxytryptamine.* London: Pergamon Press 1957, p. 87.

Benešová, O., Z. Bohdanecký, and Z. Votava: *Über einige zentrale Wirkungen von Prothiaden eines Thymolepticum aus der Reihe der 6,11-Dihydrobenz(b,c)-thiepin-Derivate.* Arzneimittel-Forsch. 14, 100—103 (1964).

Bennett, J. L., and A. K. Kooi: *Five phenothiazine derivatives: evaluation and toxicity studies.* Arch. gen. Psychiat. 4, 413—418 (1961).

Berger, F. M.: *The pharmacological properties of 2-methyl-2-n-propyl-1,3-pro-panediol dicarbamate (Miltown), a new interneuronal blocking agent.* J. Pharmacol. exp. Ther. 112, 413—423 (1954).

Bernheimer, H., W. Birkmayer u. O. Hornykiewicz: *Zur Biochemie des Parkinson-syndroms des Menschen.* Klin. Wschr. 41, 465—469 (1963).

—, u. O. Hornykiewicz: *Wirkung von Phenothiazinderivaten auf den Dopamin-(=3-Hydroxytyramin-)Stoffwechsel im Nucleus caudatus.* Naunyn-Schmiede-berg Arch. exp. Path. 251, 135 (1965).

Bertler, Å.: *Occurrence and localization of catecholamines in the human brain.* Acta physiol. scand. 51, 97—107 (1961 a).

— *Effect of reserpine on the storage of catecholamines in brain and other tissues.* Acta physiol. scand. 51, 75—83 (1961 b).

—, and E. Rosengren: *Occurrence and distribution of dopamine in brain and other tissues.* Experientia 15, 10—11 (1959).

—, N.-A. Hillarp, and E. Rosengren: *"Bound" and "free" catecholamines in the brain.* Acta physiol. scand. 50, 113—118 (1960).

— — — *Effect of reserpine on the storage of new-formed catecholamines in the adrenal medulla.* Acta physiol. scand. 52, 44—48 (1961).

Besendorf, H., u. A. Pletscher: *Beeinflussung zentraler Wirkungen von Reserpin und 5-Hydroxytryptamin durch Isonicotinsäurehydrazide.* Helv. physiol. Acta 14, 382—390 (1956).

—, F. A. Steiner, u. A. Hürlimann: *„Laroxyl", ein neues Antidepressivum mit sedierender Wirkung.* Schweiz. med. Wschr. 92, 244—246 (1962).

Bhargava, K. P., and Om. Chandra: *Tranquilizing and hypotensive activities of twelve phenothiazines.* Brit. J. Pharmacol. 22, 154—161 (1964).

—, and R. K. Srivastava: *Central effects of haloperidol on somatic reflexes.* Brit. J. Pharmacol. 25, 751—757 (1965).

Bhattacharya, B. K., and G. P. Lewis: *The effects of reserpine and compound 48/80 on the release of amines from the mast cells of rats.* Brit. J. Pharmacol. 11, 411—416 (1956).

Bianchi, C.: *Anticonvulsant action of some anti-epileptic drugs in mice pretreated with rauwolfia alkaloids.* Brit. J. Pharmacol. 11, 141—146 (1956).

Bickel, M., and M. Baggiolini: *The metabolism of imipramine and its metabolites by rat liver microsomes.* Biochem. Pharmacol. 15, 1155—1169 (1966).

Biel, J. H., A. Horita, and A. E. Drukker: *Monoamine oxidase inhibitors (hy-drazines).* In: Psychopharmacological agents, Vol. I. Ed. M. Gordon. New York-London: Academic Press 1964, pp. 359—443.

Birke, G., H. Duner, U. S. v. Euler, and L. O. Plantin: *Studies on the adreno-cortical, adreno-medullary and adrenergic nerve activity in essential hyper-tension.* Z. Vitamin-, Hormon- u. Fermentforsch. 9, 41—68 (1957).

Birkhäuser, H.: *124. Fermente im Gehirn geistig normaler Menschen (Cholinester-ase, Mono- und Diamin-oxydase, Cholin-oxydase).* Helv. chim. Acta 23, 1071 to 1086 (1940).

Birkmayer, W., u. O. Hornykiewicz: *Der L-3,4-Dihydroxyphenylalanin-(=DOPA) Effekt bei der Parkinson-Akinese.* Wien. klin. Wschr. 73, 787—788 (1961).

— — *Der L-3,4-Dioxyphenylalanin-(=DOPA)Effekt beim Parkinson-Syndrom des Menschen: Zur Pathogenese und Behandlung der Parkinson-Akinese.* Arch. Psychiat. Nervenkr., 203, 560—574 (1962).

— — *Weitere experimentelle Untersuchungen über L-DOPA beim Parkinson-Syndrom und Reserpin Parkinsonismus.* Arch. Psychiat. Nervenkr. 206, 367 to 381 (1964).

Blaschko, H.: *Amine oxidase and amine metabolism.* Pharmacol. Rev. 4, 415—458 (1952).

—, and A. D. Welch: *Localization of adrenaline in cytoplasmic particles of the bovine adrenal medulla.* Arch. exp. Path. Pharmakol. 219, 17—22 (1953).

—, G. V. R. Born, A. D'Loro, and N. R. Eade: *Observations on the distribution of catecholamines and adenosine triphosphate in the bovine adrenal medulla.* J. Physiol. 133, 548—557 (1956).

— *The development of current concepts of catecholamine formation.* Pharmacol. Rev. 11, 307—316 (1959).

—, and T. L. Chruściel: *The decarboxylation of amino acids related to tyrosine and their awakening action in reserpine-treated mice.* J. Physiol. 151, 272—284 (1960).

— *Biological inactivation by amine oxidases and time course of drug action.* Proc. 1st. int. Pharmacol. Meeting, Vol. 6. Oxford-London-New York-Paris: Perga-mon Press 1962, pp. 289—298.

Bogdanski, D. F., and S. Spector: *Comparison of central actions of cocaine and LSD.* Fed. Proc. 16, 284 (1957).

—, H. Weissbach, and S. Udenfriend: *The distribution of serotonin, 5-hydroxy-tryptophan decarboxylase and monoamine oxidase in brain.* J. Neurochem. 1, 272—278 (1957).

— — — *Pharmacological studies with the serotonin precursor, 5-hydroxytrypto-phan.* J. Pharmacol. exp. Ther. 122, 183—194 (1958).

Boissier, J.-R., and J. Pagny: *Pharmacodynamic study of a new major neuroleptic: Haloperidol (R 1625). I. Toxicity. Potentiating action of hypnosis and analgesia.* Therapie 15, 479—487 (Fr.) (1960).

— —, and Y. Font Du Picard: *Pharmacodynamic study of a new major neuroleptic: Haloperidol (R 1625). II. Sedative action at the level of the central nervous system.* Therapie 16, 279—286 (Fr.) (1961).

Bradley, P. B., and A. J. Hance: *The effect of chlorpromazine and methopromazine on the electrical activity of the brain in the cat.* Electroenceph. clin. Neuro-physiol. 9, 191—215 (1957).

—, and B. J. Key: *The effect of drugs on arousal responses produced by electrical stimulation of the reticular formation of the brain.* Electroenceph. clin. Neuro-physiol. 10, 97—110 (1958).

— — *A comparative study of the effects of drugs on the arousal system of the brain.* Brit. J. Pharmacol. 14, 340—349 (1959).

— *Phenothiazine Derivatives.* In: Physiological Pharmacology, Vol. I., Part A. Eds. W. S. Root, and F. G. Hofmann. New York-London: Academic Press 1963, pp. 417—477.

Brady, J. V.: *Assessment of drug effects on emotional behavior.* Science **123**, 1033—1034 (1956).

Brauchitsch, H.: *Endokrinologische Aspekte des Wirkungsmechanismus neuroplegischer Medikamente.* Psychopharmacologia **2**, 1—21 (1961).

Braun, G. A., G. I. Poos, and W. Soudijn: *Distribution, excretion and metabolism of neuroleptics of the butyrophenone type. Part II. Distribution, excretion and metabolism of haloperidol in Sprague-Dawley rats.* Europ. J. Pharmacol. **1**, 58—62 (1967).

Brendel W., u. H. L'Allemand: *Der Einfluß von Megaphen auf die Wärmeregulation.* Naunyn-Schmiedeberg, Arch. exp. Path. **225**, 87—89 (1955).

Brimblecombe, R. W., and A. L. Green: *Effect of monoamine oxidase inhibitors on the behavior of rats in Hall's open field.* Nature **194**, 983 (1962).

Brodie, B. B., P. A. Shore, and S. L. Silver: *Potentiating action of chlorpromazine and reserpine.* Nature, **175**, 1133—1134 (1955).

—, A. Pletscher, and P. A. Shore: *Possible role of serotonin in brain function and in reserpine action.* J. Pharmacol. exp. Ther., **116**, 9 (1956 a).

—, P. A. Shore, and A. Pletscher: *Serotonin releasing activity limited to rauwolfia alkaloids with tranquilizing action.* Science **123**, 992—993 (1956 b).

—, E. G. Tomich, R. Kuntzmann, and P. A. Shore: *On the mechanism of action of reserpine: effect of reserpine on capacity of tissues to bind serotonin.* J. Pharmacol. exp. Ther. **119**, 461—467 (1957).

—, S. Spector, and P. A. Shore: *Interaction of drugs with norepinephrine in the brain.* Pharmacol. Rev. **11**, 548—564 (1959 a).

— — — *Interaction of monoamine oxidase inhibitors with physiological and biochemical mechanisms in brain.* Ann. N. Y. Acad. Sci. **80**, 609—616 (1959 b).

—, K. F. Finger, F. B. Orlans, G. P. Quinn, and F. Sulser: *Evidence that tranquilizing action of reserpine is associated with changes in brain serotonin and not in brain norepinephrine.* J. Pharmacol. exp. Ther., **129**, 250—256 (1960).

—, R. P. Maickel, and E. O. Westermann: *Action of reserpine on pituitary-adrenocortical system through possible action on hypothalamus.* In: Regional neurochemistry. Eds. S. S. Kety and I. Elkes. Oxford-London-New York-Paris: Pergamon Press 1961 a, pp. 351—361.

—, M. H. Bickel, and F. Sulser: *Desmethylimipramine, a new type of antidepressant drug.* Med. exp. **5**, 454—458 (1961 b).

—, and E. Costa: *Some current views on brain monoamines.* In: Monoamines et système nerveux central. Symposium Bel-Air. Ed. J. de Ajuriaguerra. Geneve: Georg et Cie; Paris: Masson et Cie 1962, pp. 13—49.

—, and M. Beavan: *Neurochemical transducer systems.* Med. exp. **8**, 320—351 (1963).

Brook, G. W.: *Withdrawal from neuroleptic drugs.* Amer. J. Psychiat. **115**, 931 to 932 (1959).

Brücke, F. Th.: *Beiträge zur Pharmakologie des Bulbocapnins.* Naunyn-Schmiedeberg Arch. exp. Path. **179**, 504—523 (1935).

— *Das Wesen der Bulbocapnin-starre.* Naunyn-Schmiedeberg Arch. exp. Path. **182**, 325—330 (1936).

—, H. Petsche, S. Sailer u. Ch. Stumpf: *Apomorphinwirkung auf das Kaninchen-EEG.* Naunyn-Schmiedeberg Arch. exp. Path. **230**, 335—346 (1957 a).

—, S. Sailer u. Ch. Stumpf: *Pharmakologische Beeinflussung der Frequenz der Hippocampustätigkeit während retikularer Reizung.* Naunyn-Schmiedeberg Arch. exp. Path. Pharmak. **231**, 267—278 (1957 b).

— — — *Wechselwirkung zwischen Physostigmin einerseits und Evipan, Procain, Largactil und Scopolamin andererseits auf die rhinencephale Tätigkeit des Kaninchens.* Naunyn-Schmiedeberg Arch. exp. Path. **232**, 433—441 (1958).

Brücke, F. Th., and G. Spring: *Über die Wirkung sympathicotroper Stoffe auf den Schließmuskel der Kardia.* Naunyn-Schmiedeberg Arch. exp. Path. 245, 374 bis 382 (1963).

—, u. Ch. Stumpf: Unveröffentlichte Befunde.

Brune, G. G., T. Kobayashi, C. Bull, T. T. Tourlentes, and H. E. Himwich. *Relevance of drug-induced extrapyramidal reactions to behavioral changes during neuroleptic treatment. II. Combined treatment with trifluoperazine-amobarbital.* Comprehens. Psychiat. 3, 292—296 (1962 a).

—, C. Morpurgo, A. Bielkus, T. Kobayashi, T. T. Tourlentes, and H. E. Himwich: *Relevance of drug-induced extrapyramidal reactions to behavioral changes during neuroleptic treatment. I. Treatment with trifluoperazine singly and in combination with trihexyphenidyl.* Comprehens. Psychiat. 3, 228—234 (1962 b).

Buffoni, F., and H. Blaschko: *Benzylamineoxidase and histaminase: purification and crystallization of an enzyme from pig plasma.* Proc. roy. Soc. Biol. 161, 153—167 (1964).

— *Histaminase and related amine oxidases.* Pharmacol. Rev. 18, 1163—1199 (1966).

Burack, W. R., N. Weiner, and P. B. Hagen: *The effect of reserpine on the catecholamine and adenine nucleotide contents of adrenal gland.* J. Pharmacol. exp. Ther. 130, 245—250 (1960).

Burge, E: *Einfluß von Tranquilizer-Substanzen auf die Alkoholwirkung.* Hefte Unfallheilk. 24, 99—102 (1961).

Burger, M.: *Veränderungen der Adrenalin- und Noradrenalinkonzentration im menschlichen Blutplasma unter Reserpin.* Naunyn-Schmiedeberg Arch. exp. Path. 230, 489—498 (1957).

Burke, J. C., G. L. Hassert jr., and J. P. High: *The tranquilizing activity of 10-(3-dimethylaminopropyl)-2-(trifluoromethyl)-phenothiazine hydrochloride (MC 4703) and related phenothiazines in animal.* J. Pharmacol. exp. Ther. 119, 136 (1957).

Burkman, A. M.: *Potent anti-apomorphine action of fluophenazine in pigeons.* Arch. int. Pharmacodyn. 137, 396—403 (1962).

Burn, J. H., and R. Hobbs: *A test for tranquilizing drugs.* Arch. int. Pharmacodyn. 113, 290—295 (1957).

—, and M. J. Rand: *The action of sympathomimetic amines in animals treated with reserpine.* J. Physiol. 144, 314—336 (1958).

— — *The cause of the supersensitivity of smooth muscle to noradrenaline after sympathetic degeneration.* J. Physiol. 147, 135—143 (1959).

— *Tyramine and other amines are noradrenaline-releasing substances.* In: Adrenergic mechanisms. Eds. J. R. Vane, G. E. W. Wolstenholme, and J. O'Connor. London: Pub. J. & A. Churchill 1960, pp. 326—336.

Cairncross, K. D.: *On the peripheral pharmacology of amitriptyline.* Arch. int. Pharmacodyn. 154, 438—448 (1965).

Callingham, B. A., and M. Mann: *Depletion and replacement of the adrenaline and noradrenaline contents of the rat adrenal gland, following treatment with reserpine.* Brit. J. Pharmacol. 18, 138—149 (1962).

Cammanni, F., O. Losana, and G. M. Molinatti: *Selective depletion of noradrenaline in the adrenal medulla of the rat after administration of reserpine.* Experientia 14, 199—201 (1958).

—, G. M. Molinatti, and M. Olivetti: *Abolitisn by chlorpromazine of the inhibiting effect of iproniazid on the depletion of adrenal catecholamines induced by reserpine.* Nature 184, 65—66 (1959).

Campos, H. A., and F. E. Shideman: *Subcellular distribution of catecholamines in the dog heart. Effects of reserpine and norepinephrine administration.* Int. J. Neuropharmacol. 1, 13—22 (1962).

Carlsson, A, and N.-A. Hillarp: *Release of adrenaline from the adrenal medulla of rabbits produced by reserpine.* Kungl. Fysiogr. Sällsk. Förhandl., 26, 1—2 (1956).

—, M. Lindqvist, and T. Magnusson: *3,4-Dihydroxyphenylalanine and 5-hydroxytryptophan as reserpine antagonists.* Nature 180, 1200 (1957 a).

—, E. Rosengren, A. Bertler, and J. Nilsson: *Effect of reserpine on the metabolism of catecholamines.* In: Psychotropic drugs. Eds. S. Garattini, and V. Ghetti. Amsterdam: Elsevier Publ. Co. 1957 b, pp. 363—372.

—, M. Lindqvist, T. Magnusson, and B. Waldeck: *On the presence of 3-hydroxytyramine in brain.* Science, 127, 471 (1958).

— — — *The effect of monoamine oxidase inhibitors on the metabolism of the brain catecholamines.* In: Simposio international sobre nialamida. J. Soc. Cienc. Med. Lisboa 123, Suppl. (1959 a), pp. 96—98.

—, E. B. Rasmussen, and P. Kristjansen: *The urinary excretion of adrenaline and noradrenaline by schizophrenic patients during reserpine treatment.* J. Neurochem. 4, 318—320 (1959 b).

— *The occurrence, distribution and physiological role of catecholamines in the nervous system.* Pharmacol. Rev. 11, 490—493 (1959).

—, M. Lindqvist, and T. Magnusson: *On the biochemistry and possible functions of dopamine and noradrenaline in brain.* In: Adrenergic mechanisms. Eds. J. R. Vane, G. E. W. Wostenholme, and M. O'Connor. London: J. & A. Churchill, Ltd. 1960, pp. 432—439.

— *Brain monoamines and psychotropic drugs.* In: Neuropsychopharmacology, Vol 2. Ed. E. Rothlin. Amsterdam-London-New York-Princeton: Elsevier Publ. Co. 1961, pp. 417—421.

—, N.-A. Hillarp, and B. Waldeck: *A Mg^{++}-ATP dependent storage mechanism in the amine granules of the adrenal medulla.* Med. exp. 6, 47—53 (1962).

—, and M. Lindqvist: *Effect of chlorpromazine or haloperidol on formation of 3-methoxytyramine and normetanephrine in mouse brain.* Acta Pharmacol. Toxicol. 20, 140—144 (1963).

— *Functional significance of drug-induced changes in brain monoamine levels.* In: Progress in drug research, biogenic amines, Vol. 8. Eds. H. E. Himwich, and W. A. Himwich. Amsterdam-London-New York: Elsevier Publ. Co. 1964, p. 14.

—, and B. Waldeck: *Inhibition of H^3-Metaraminol uptake by antidepressive and related agents.* J. Pharm. Pharmacol. 17, 243—244 (1965).

Carlton, P. L.: *Potentiation of the behavioral effects of amphetamine by imipramine.* Psychopharmacologia 2, 364—376 (1961).

Cassano, G. B., and E. Hansson: *Autoradiographic distribution studies in mice with C^{14}-imipramine.* Int. J. Neuropsychiat. 2 (3), 269—278 (1966).

Chen, G., and C. R. Ensor: *Antagonism studies on reserpine and certain CNS depressants.* Proc. Soc. exp. Biol. Med. 87, 602—608 (1954).

— —, and B. Bohner: *A facilitation action of reserpine on the central nervous system.* Proc. Soc. exp. Biol. Med. 86, 507—510 (1954).

Chessin, M., B. Dubnick, E. R. Kramer, and C. C. Scott: *Modifications of pharmacology of reserpine and serotonin by iproniazid.* Fed. Proc. 15, 409 (1956).

—, E. R. Kramer, and C. C. Scott: *Modifications of the pharmacology of reserpine and serotonin by iproniazid.* J. Pharmacol. exp. Ther. 119, 453—460 (1957).

Cheymol, J., et C. Levassort: *Hyperthermisant et chlorpromazine.* C. R. Soc. Biol. 149, 475—480 (1955).

Chow, M., and C. D. Hendley: *Effect of monoamine oxidase inhibitors on experimental convulsions.* Fed. Proc. 18, 376 (1959).

Christensen, J., and A. W. Wase: *Distribution of S³⁵ in the mouse after administration of S³⁵ 10(dimethylaminopropyl)-2-chlorophenothiazine (chlorpromazine).* Acta Pharmacol. Toxicol. 12, 81—84 (1956).

Chusid, J. G., L. M. Kopeloff, and N. Kopeloff: *Reserpine (Serpasil) effects on epileptic monkeys.* Proc. Soc. exp. Biol. Med. 88, 276—277 (1955).

— — *Chlordiazepoxide as an anticonvulsant in monkeys.* Proc. Soc. exp. Biol. Med. 109, 546—548 (1962).

Clark, M. L., and P. C. Johnson: *Amenorrhea and elevated level of serum cholesterol produced by a trifluomethylated phenothiazine (SKF-5354-A).* J. clin. Endocrinol. 20, 641—646 (1960).

Cole, H. F., and H. H. Wolf: *The effects of some psychotropic drugs on conditioned avoidance and aggressive behaviors.* Psychopharmacologia 8, 389—396 (1966).

Cole, J., and P. Glees: *Ritalin as an antagonist to reserpine in monkeys.* Lancet 1, 338 (1956).

Cole, J. O., and D. J. Clyde: cit. Toman, J. E. P.

Consolo, S., E. Dolfini, S. Garattini, and L. Valzelli: *Desipramine and amphetamine metabolism.* J. Pharm. Pharmacol. 19, 253—256 (1967).

Cook, L., and R. T. Kelleher: *Drug effects on the behavior of animals.* Ann. N. Y. Acad. Sci. 96, 315—335 (1962).

— — *Effect of drugs on behavior.* Ann. Rev. Pharmacol. 3, 205—222 (1963).

—, and J. J. Toner: *The antiemetic action of chlorpromazine, SKF 2601-A (RP 4560).* J. Pharmacol. exp. Ther. 110, 12 (1954).

—, and E. Weidley: *Behavioral effects of some psychopharmacological agents.* Ann. N. Y. Acad. Sci. 66, 740—752 (1957).

Costa, E., G. R. Pscheidt, W. G. Van Meter, and H. E. Himwich: *Brain concentrations biogenic amines and EEG patterns of rabbits.* J. Pharmacol. exp. Ther. 130, 81—88 (1960).

Coupland, R. E.: *Strain sensitivity of albino rats to reserpine.* Nature 181, 930 to 931 (1958).

Courvoisier, S., J. Fournel, R. Ducrot, M. Kolsky, et P. Koetschet: *Propriétés pharmacodynamiques du chlorhydrate de chloro-3(dimethyl-amino-3'-propyl)-10 Phénothiazine (4.560 R. P.).* Arch. int. Pharmacodyn. 92, 305—361 (1953).

—, R. Ducrot, J. Fournel et L. Julou: *Propriétés pharmacodynamiques de la méthopromazine, nouveau neuroleptique apparenté a la chlorpromazine.* C. R. Soc. Biol. 151, 689—692 (1957 a).

— — — — *Propriétés pharmacodynamique générales de la lévomépromazine (7.044 R. P.).* C. R. Soc. Biol. 151, 1378—1382 (1957 b).

— — — — *Propriétés pharmacodynamiques générales de la prochlorpémazine (6.140 R. P.).* C. R. Soc. Biol. 151, 1144—1148 (1957 c).

— — et L. Julou: *Nouveaux aspects expérimentaux de l'activité centrale des dérivés de la phénothiazine.* In: Psychotropic drugs. Eds. S. Garattini and V. Ghetti. Amsterdam: Elsevier Publ. Co. 1957 d, pp. 373—391.

— —, J. Fournel et L. Julou: *Propriétés pharmacologiques générales d'un nouveau dérivé de la phénothiazine, neuroleptique puissant a action neurovégétative discrete, le chlorhydrate de (méthyl-2'-diméthylamino-3'-propyl-1')-10 phénothiazine (6.549 R. P.).* Arch. int. Pharmacodyn. 115, 90—113 (1958).

Creveling, C. R., J. Daly, T. Tokuyama, and B. Witkop: *The combined use of α-methyltyrosine and threo-dihydroxyphenylserine-selective reduction of dopamine levels in the central nervous system.* Biochem.Pharmacol. 17, 65—70 (1968).

Cronheim, G., and I. M. Toekes: *Comparison of some pharmacological properties of rescinnamine and reserpine, two alkaloids isolated from Rauwolfia serpentina.* J. Pharmacol. exp. Ther. 113, 13 (1955).

Crout, J. R., C. R. Creveling, and S. Udenfriend: *Norepinephrine metabolism in rat brain and heart.* J. Pharmacol. exp. Ther. 132, 269—277 (1961).

—, A. J. Muskus, and U. Trendelenburg: *Effect of tyramine on isolated guineapig atria in relation to their noradrenaline stores.* Brit. J. Pharmacol. 18, 600—611 (1962).

Curzon, G.: *The biochemistry of dyskinesias.* Eds. C. C. Pfeiffer and J. R. Smythies. Int. Review Neurobiol. 10, 323—370 (1967).

DaPrada, M., and A. Pletscher: *Acceleration of the cerebral dopamine turnover by chlorpromazine.* Experientia (Basel) 22, 465—466 (1966).

Das, N. N., S. R. Dasgupta, and G. Werner: *Changes of behavior and EEG in rhesus monkeys caused by chlorpromazine.* Arch. int. Pharmacodyn. 99, 451 to 457 (1954).

Dasgupta, S. R., and G. Werner: *Inhibition of hypothalamic, medullary and reflex vasomotor responses by chlorpromazine.* Brit. J. Pharmacol. 9, 389—391 (1954).

—, K. L. Mukherje, and G. Werner: *The activity of some central depressant drugs in acute decorticate and diencephalic preparations.* Arch. int. Pharmacodyn. 97, 149—156 (1954).

—, and G. Werner: *Inhibitory actions of chlorpromazine on motor activity.* Arch. in. Pharmacodyn. 100, 409—417 (1955).

— cit. E. K. Killam (1962).

Davidson, A. N.: *Physiological role of monoamine oxidase.* Physiol. Rev. 38, 729—747 (1958).

Dawkins, M. J. R., J. D. Judah, and K. R. Rees: *The effect of chlorpromazine on the respiratory chain.* Biochem. J. 72, 204—209 (1959).

De Feo, V. J., and S. R. M. Reynolds: *Modification of the menstrual cycle in the rhesus monkey by reserpine.* Science 124, 726—727 (1956).

— *Effect of large doses of reserpine on the deciduoma response.* Anat. Rec. 127, 409 (1957).

Degkwitz, R., R. Frowein, C. Kulenkampff u. U. Mohs: *Über die Wirkungen des L-DOPA beim Menschen und deren Beeinflussung durch Reserpin, Chlorpromazin, Iproniazid und Vitamin B_6.* Klin. Wschr. 38, 120—123 (1960).

—, u. O. Luxenburger: *Das terminale extrapyramidale Insuffizienz- bzw. Defektsyndrom infolge chronischer Anwendung von Neurolepticis.* Nervenarzt. 36, 173—175 (1965).

De Jong, H., et H. Buruk: *La Catatonie experimentale par la bulbocapnine.* In: Etude physiologique et clinique. Paris: Masson et Cie 1930.

De Jongh, D. K., and E. G. Van Proosdij-Hartzema: *Investigations into experimental hypertension.* IV. Acta Physiol. Pharmacol. Neerl. 4, 175—186 (1955).

Delay, J. F., et P. Deniker: *Trente-huit cas de psychoses traitées par la cure prolongée et continué de 4560 R. P.* In: C. R. due Congres des Al. et Neurol. de Langue Fr. Paris: Masson et Cie 1952.

— — et J. M. Harl: *Utilization en therapeutique psychiatrique d'une phenothiazine d'action centrale elective (4560 R. P.).* Ann. Medicopsychol. 110, 112—117 (1952).

Delga, J., et R. Hazard: *Action de la chlorpromazine sur quelques action de l'adrenaline et de la noradrenaline chez le chien.* Arch. int. Pharmacodyn. 109, 446—456 (1957).

Delgado, M. M. R., and L. Mihailovic: *Use of intracerebral electrodes to evaluate drugs that act on the central nervous system.* Ann. N. Y. Acad. Sci. 64, 644—666 (1956).

De Long, S. J., B. J. Poley, J. R. McFarlane, Jr.: *Ocular changes associated with long-term chlorpromazine therapy.* Arch. Ophthalm. (Chicago) 73, 611—617 (1965).

De Maar, E. W. J., W. R. Martin, and K. R. Unna: *Chlorpromazine II: The effects of chlorpromazine on evoked potentials in the midbrain reticular formation.* J. Pharmacol. exp. Ther. 124, 77—85 (1958).

Dengler, H. J., u. E. O. Titus: *Die Aufnahme von H^3-Noradrenalin in Gewebe-Schnitte und deren Beeinflussung durch Pharmaka.* Naunyn-Schmiedeberg Arch. exp. Path. 241, 523 (1961).

—, I. A. Michaelson, H. E. Spiegel, and E. Titus: *The uptake of labeled norepinephrine by isolated brain and other tissues of the cat.* Int. J. Neuropharmacol. 1, 12—38 (1962).

Dennison, A. D., P. T. White, R. B. Moore, and W. J. Pierce: *Effect of reserpine upon the human electroencephalogram.* Neurology 5, 56—58 (1955).

Desci, L.: *Further studies on the metabolic background of tranquilizing drug action.* Psychopharmacologia 2, 224—242 (1961).

Dews, P. B., and W. H. Morse: *Behavioral pharmacology.* Ann. Rev. Pharmacol. 1, 145—174 (1961).

Diassi, P. A., F. L. Weisenborn, C. M. Dylion, and O. Wintersteiner: *On the sterochemistry of reserpine.* J. Amer. Chem. Soc. 77, 4687—4688 (1955).

Dingell, J. V., F. Sulser, and J. R. Gillette: *Species differences in the metabolism of imipramine and desmethylimipramine (DMI).* J. Pharmacol. exp. Ther. 143, 14—22 (1964).

Dobkin, A., R. G. B. Gilbert, and K. I. Melville: cit. W. F. T. Tatlow, C. M. Fischer, and A. B. Dobkin: *The clinical effects of chlorpromazine on dyskinesia.* Canad. med. Ass. 71, 380—381 (1954).

Domenjoz, R., u. W. Theobald: *Zur Pharmakologie des Tofranil® (N-[3-Di-methylaminopropyl]-iminodibenzyl-hydrochloride).* Arch. int. Pharmacodyn. 120, 450—489 (1959).

Domino, E. F., and R. H. Rech: *Differences in the blood pressure response to reserpine on anaesthetized and unanaesthetized dogs immobilized with neuro-muscular blocking agents.* J. Pharmacol. exp. Ther. 119, 142—143 (1957).

— *Sites of action of some central nervous system depressants.* Ann. Rev. Pharmacol. 2, 215—250 (1962 a).

— *Human pharmacology of tranquilizing drugs.* Clin. Pharmacol. Ther. 3, 599—664 (1962 b).

— *Centrally acting skeletal muscle relaxants.* In: Pharmacometrics. Eds. D. R. Laurence and A. L. Bacharach. New York: Academic Press 1964, pp. 313—324.

Dresse, A., and R. De Meyer: *Influence of four butyrophenone neuroleptics on rat brain noradrenaline depletory effect of reserpine.* Life Sci. 3, 759—762 (1964).

— *Influence of 15 neuroleptics (butyrophenones and phenothiazines) on rat brain noradrenaline and self-stimulation behavior.* Arch. int. Pharmacodyn. 159, 353—365 (1966).

Dreyfuss, F.: *Jaundice due to chlorpromazine.* J. Amer. med. Ass. 168, 2044 (1958).

Druckman, R., D. Seelinger, and G. Thulin: *Chronic involuntary movements induced by phenothiazines.* J. nerv. ment. Dis. 135, 69—76 (1962).

Dubnick, B., G. A. Leeson, and G. E. Phillips: *An effect of monoamine oxidase inhibitors on brain serotonin of mice in addition to that resulting from inhibition of monoamine oxidase.* J. Neurochem. 9, 299—306 (1962).

Dubnick, B., D. F. Morgan, and G. E. Philipps: *Inhibition of monoamine oxidase by 2-methyl-3-piperidino-pyrazine.* Ann. N. Y. Acad. Sci. 107, 914—922 (1963).

Efron, D. H., and G. L. Gessa: *Failure of ethanol and barbiturates to alter brain monoamine content.* Arch. int. Pharmacodyn. 142, 111—116 (1963).

Egdahl, R. H., J. B. Richards, and D. M. Hume: *Effect of reserpine on adrenocortical function of unanesthetized dogs.* Science 123, 418 (1956).

Ehringer, H., u. O. Hornykiewicz: *Verteilung von Noradrenalin und Dopamin (3-Hydroxytyramin) im Gehirn des Menschen und ihr Verhalten bei Erkrankungen des extrapyramidalen Systems.* Klin. Wschr. 38, 1236—1239 (1960).

— — u. K. Lechner: *Die Wirkung des Chlorpromazins auf den Katecholamin- und 5-Hydroxytryptaminstoffwechsel im Gehirn der Ratte.* Naunyn-Schmiedeberg Arch. exp. Path. 239, 507—519 (1960).

— — — *Die Wirkung von Methylenblau auf die Monoaminoxydase und den Katecholamin- und 5-Hydroxytryptaminstoffwechsel des Gehirnes.* Naunyn-Schmiedeberg Arch. exp. Path. 241, 568—582 (1961).

Eichler-Satke, I.: *Über die Wirkung der Phenothiazinderivate.* Subsidia med. (Wien) 10, 43—69 (1958).

Eidelberg, E., H. M. Neer, and M. K. Miller: *Anticonvulsant properties of some benzodiazepine derivatives: Possible use against psychomotor seizures.* Neurology 15, 223—230 (1965).

Eltherington, L. G., and A. Horita: *Some pharmacological actions of β-phenyl-isopropylhydrazine (PIH).* J. Pharmacol. exp. Ther. 128, 7—14 (1960).

Emås, S.: *Gastric acid secretion in gastric fistula cats during reserpine treatment.* Acta. Physiol. scand. 59, 169—183 (1963).

Emele, J. F., J. Shanaman, and M. R. Warren: *The analgesic activity of phenelzine and other compounds.* J. Pharmacol. exp. Ther. 134, 206—209 (1961).

Eranko, O., and V. Hopsu: *Effect of reserpine on the histochemistry and content of adrenaline and noradrenaline in the adrenal medulla of the rat and the mouse.* Endocrinology 62, 15—23 (1958).

Esplin, D. W., and D. G. Heaton: *Effect of reserpine on spinal cord synaptic transmission.* J. Pharmacol. exp. Ther. 121, 267—271 (1957).

von Euler, U. S., and A. Purkhold: *Effect of sympathetic denervation on the noradrenaline and adrenaline content of the spleen, kidney and salivary glands in the sheep.* Acta Physiol. scand. 24, 212—217 (1951).

—, and S. Hellner-Bjorkman: *Effect of amine oxidase inhibitors on noradrenaline and adrenaline content of cat organs.* Acta Physiol. scand. 33 (Suppl. 118), 21—25 (1955).

—, and N.-A. Hillarp: *Evidence for the presence of noradrenaline in submicrosopic structures of adrenergic axone.* Nature 177, 44—45 (1956).

—, and F. Lishajko: *Effect of reserpine on the uptake of catecholamines in isolated nerve storage granules.* Int. J. Neuropharmacol. 2, 127—134 (1963).

Everett, G. M., J. E. P. Toman, and A. H. Smith, Jr.: *Reduction of electroshock latency and other central actions of reserpine.* Fed. Proc. 14, 337 (1955).

— — — *Central and peripheral effects of reserpine and 11-desmethoxyreserpine (harmonyl) on the nervous system.* Fed. Proc. 16, 1263 (1957).

—, J. C. David, and J. E. P. Toman: *Pharmacological studies of monoamine oxidase inhibitors.* Fed. Proc. 18, 388 (1959).

— *Some electrophysiological and biochemical correlates of motor activity and aggressive behavior.* In: Neuropsychopharmacology, Vol. 2. Ed. E. Rothlin. Amsterdam-London-New York-Princeton: Elsevier Publ. Co. 1961, pp. 379 to 384.

Everett, G. M., and R. G. Wiegand: *Non-hydrazide monoamine oxidase inhibitors and their effects on central amines and motor behavior.* Biochem. Pharmacol. 8, 163 (1961).

— — *Central amines and behavioral states: a critique and new data.* Proc. 1st. int. Pharmacol. Meeting, Vol. 8. Oxford-London-New York-Paris: Pergamon Press 1962, pp. 85—92.

— *The DOPA response potentiation test and its use in screening for antidepressant drugs.* In: Antidepressant drugs. Eds. S. Garattini and M. N. G. Dukes. Amsterdam: Excerpta Medica Fdn. 1967, pp. 164—167.

Feldberg, W., and R. D. Myers: *A new concept of temperature regulation by amines in the hypothalamus.* Nature 200, 1325 (1963).

— — *Effects on temperature of amines injected into the cerebral ventricles. A new concept of temperature regulation.* J. Physiol. 173, 226—237 (1964).

Fellows, E. J., and L. Cook: *The comparative pharmacology of a number of phenothiazine derivatives.* In: Psychotropic drugs. Eds. S. Garattini and V. Ghetti. Amsterdam-London-New York-Princeton: Elsevier Publ. Co. 1957, pp. 397—404.

Fischbach, R., G. Harrer u. H. Harrer: *Verstärkung der Noradrenalin-Wirkung durch Psychopharmaka beim Menschen.* Arzneimittel-Forschung 2, 263—265 (1966).

Fischer, J. E., W. D. Horst, and I. J. Kopin: *β-Hydroxylated sympathomimetic amines as false neurotransmitters.* Brit. J. Pharmacol. 24, 477—484 (1965 a).

—, I. J. Kopin, and J. Axelrod: *Evidence for extraneuronal binding of norepinephrine.* J. Pharmacol. exp. Ther. 147, 181—185 (1965 b).

Fleming, W. W., and U. Trendelenburg: *The development of supersensitivity to norepinephrine after pretreatment with reserpine.* J. Pharmacol. exp. Ther. 133, 41—51 (1961).

Folkerts, J., and E. Spiegel: *Tremor on stimulation of the midbrain tegmentum.* Confin. Neurol. 13, 193—202 (1953).

Freeman, A. R., and M. A. Spirtes: *Effects of chlorpromazine on biological membranes. II. Chlorpromazine-induced changes in human erythrocytes.* Biochem. Pharmacol. 12, 47—53 (1963).

Friebel, H., u. C. Reichle: *Zur analgetischen und analgesieverstärkenden Wirkung von Chlorpromazin (Megaphen).* Naunyn-Schmiedeberg Arch. exp. Path. 226, 551—557 (1955).

Friedhoff, A. J., L. Hekimian, M. Alpert, and E. Tobach: *Dihydroxyphenylalanine in extrapyramidal disease.* J. Amer. med. Ass. 184, 285—286 (1963).

Friend, O. G., M. S. Zileli, J. T. Hamlin, and F. J. Reuter: cit. A. Pletscher, K. F. Gey, and P. Zeller.

Frommel, E., C. Fleury, J. Schmidt-Ginzkey, and M. Beguin: *The psychotropic action of atropine and scopolamine and their position in psychopharmacology: an experimental study.* Arzneimittel-Forsch. 12, 309—314 (1962).

—, I. V. Ledebur, and M. Beguin: *De l'antagonisme de la nalorphine envers la chlorpromazine. Etude experimentale d'antidotisme.* Arch. int. Pharmacodyn. 143, 52—77 (1963).

— —, and J. Seydoux: *Study of the effects of morphine and nalorphine.* Arch. int. Pharmacodyn. 152, 144—155 (1964).

—, and M. Chmouliovsky: *The antagonism of haloperidol to amphetamine in the mouse (Fr.).* C. R. Soc. Biol. 158, 48—50 (1964).

Funderburk, W. H., K. F. Finger, A. B. Drakontides, and J. A. Schneider: *EEG and biochemical findings with MAO inhibitors.* Ann. N. Y. Acad. Sci. 96, 289—301 (1962).

Fuxe, K., and U. Ungerstedt: *Localization of 5-hydroxytryptamine uptake in rat brain after intraventricular injection.* J. Pharm. Pharmacol. 19, 335—337 (1967).
— *Serotonin-LSD interactions.* Ann. N. Y. Acad. Sci. 66, 643—647 (1957).

Gaddum, J. H., and K. A. Hameed: *Drugs which antagonize 5-hydroxytryptamine.* Brit. J. Pharmacol. 9, 240—248 (1954).
—, W. A. Krovoy, and S. G. Laverty: *The action of reserpine on the excretion of adrenaline and noradrenaline.* J. Neurochem. 2, 249—253 (1958).

Gaffney, T. E., D. H. Morrow, and C. A. Chidsey: *The role of myocardial catecholamines in the response to tyramine.* J. Pharmacol. exp. Ther. 137, 301—305 (1962).

Gangloff, H., u. M. Monnier: *Topische Bestimmung des zerebralen Angriffs von Reserpin (Serpasil).* Experientia 11, 404—407 (1955).
— — *Topic action of reserpine, serotonin and chlorpromazine on the unanesthetized rabbit's brain.* Helv. physiol. Acta 15, 83—104 (1957).

Garattini, S., A. Giachetti, A. Jori, L. Pieri, and L. Valzelli: *Effect of imipramine, amitriptyline and their monomethyl derivatives on reserpine activity.* J. Pharm. Pharmacol. 14, 509—514 (1962).

Gatti, C. L.: *Azione dei farmaci tranquillanti sui vari tipi di comportamento del ratto condizionato.* In: Psychotropic drugs. Eds. S. Garattini and V. Ghetti. Amsterdam: Elsevier Publ. Co. 1957, pp. 125—135.

Gaunt, R., A. A. Renzi, N. Antouchak, G. J. Miller, and M. Gilman: *Endocrine aspects of the pharmacology of reserpine.* Ann. N. Y. Acad. Sci. 59, 22—35 (1954).
—, J. J. Chart, and A. A. Renzi: *Endocrine pharmacology.* Science 133, 613—621 (1961).

Geller, I., J. T. Kolak, Jr., and J. Seifter: *The effects of chlordiazepoxide and chlorpromazine on a punishment discrimination.* Psychopharmacologia 3, 374—385 (1962).

Gerstenbrand, F., u. K. Pateisky: *Über die Wirkung von L-DOPA auf die motorischen Störungen beim Parkinson-Syndrom.* Wien. Z. Nervenheilk. 20, 90—100 (1962).
— — u. P. Prosenz: *Erfahrungen mit L-DOPA in der Therapie des Parkinsonismus.* Psychiat. Neurol. 146, 246—261 (1963).

Gertner, S. B., M. K. Paasonen, and N. J. Giarman: *Presence of 5-hydroxytryptamine (serotonin) in perfusate from sympathetic ganglia.* Fed. Proc. 16, 299 (1957).
— *The effects of monoamine oxidase inhibitors on ganglionic transmission.* J. Pharmacol. exp. Ther. 131, 223—230 (1961).

Gessa, G. L., E. Cuenca, and E. Costa: *On the mechanism of hypotensive effects of MAO-inhibitors.* Ann. N. Y. Acad. Sci. 107, 935—941 (1963).

Gey, K. F., u. A. Pletscher: *Vermehrung der Serum-Milchsäure durch Monoaminoxidase-Hemmer.* Helv. physiol. pharmacol. Acta 18, C 70—C 73 (1960).
— — *Einfluß von Chlorpromazine und Chlorprothixen auf den Monoamin-Stoffwechsel des Rattenhirns.* Helv. physiol. pharmacol. Acta 19, C 22—C 24 (1961 a).
— — *Influence of chlorpromazine and chlorprothixene on the cerebral metabolism of 5-hydroxytryptamine, norepinephrine and dopamine.* J. Pharmacol. exp. Ther. 133, 18—24 (1961 b).
— — *Activity of monoamine oxidase in relation to the 5-hydroxytryptamine and norepinephrine content of the rat brain.* J. Neurochem. 6, 239—243 (1961 c).
—, W. P. Burkard, and A. Pletscher: *Influence of chlorpromazine on decarboxylases of aromatic amino acids.* Biochem. Pharmacol. 8, 383—387 (1961).

131

Gey, K. F., and A. Pletscher: *Interference of chlorpromazine with the metabolism of aromatic amino acids in rat brain.* Nature 194, 387—389 (1962 a).

— — *Effect of α-alkylated tryptamine derivatives on 5-hydroxytryptamine metabolism in vivo.* Brit. J. Pharmacol. 19, 161—167 (1962 b).

— —, and W. Burkard: *Effect of inhibitors of monoamine oxidase on various enzymes and on the storage of monoamines.* Ann. N. Y. Acad. Sci. 107, 1147—1151 (1963).

— — *Effecas of chlorpromazine on the metabolism of dl-2-C¹⁴-DOPA in the rat.* J. Pharmacol. exp. Ther. 145, 337—343 (1964).

Giarman, N. J., and S. Schanberg: *The intracellular distribution of 5-hydroxy-tryptamine (HT; serotonin) in the rat's brain.* Biochem. Pharmacol. 1, 301—306 (1958).

Gillette, J. R., J. V. Dingell, F. Sulser, R. Kuntzman, and B. B. Brodie: *Isolation from rat brain of a metabolic product, desmethylimipramine, that mediates the antidepressant activity of imipramine (Tofranil).* Experientia 17, 417—418 (1961).

Glowinski, J., and J. Axelrod: *Inhibition of uptake of tritiated noradrenaline in the intact rat brain by imipramine and structurally related compounds.* Nature 204, 1318—1319 (1964).

— —, and L. L. Iverson: *Regional studies of catecholamines in the rat brain.* J. Pharmacol. exp. Ther. 153, 30—41 (1966).

Gluckman, M. I.: *Pharmacology of oxazepam (Serax), a new antianxiety agent.* Curr. Ther. Pres. 7, 721—740 (1965).

Goldberg, L. L., and F. M. Da Costa: *Selective depression of sympathetic transmission by intravenous administration of iproniazid and harmine.* Proc. Soc. exp. Biol. Med. 105, 223—227 (1960).

Goldberg, N. D., and F. E. Shideman: *Species differences in the cardiac effects of a monoamine oxidase inhibitor.* J. Pharmacol. exp. Ther. 136, 142—151 (1962).

Goldman, D.: cit. E. F. Domino (1962 b).

Goldstein, M., A. J. Friedhoff, and G. Sandler: *The relative metabolic rates of norepinephrine-7-H³ and epinephrine-1-C¹⁴.* Experientia 16, 211 (1960).

—, and J. M. Musacchio: *Effects of monoamine oxidase inhibition on biogenic amine metabolism.* Ann. N. Y. Acad. Sci. 107, 840—847 (1963).

Goodall, Mc. C.: *Studies on noradrenaline and adrenaline in mammalian heart.* Acta Physiol. scand. 24 (Suppl.), 85 (1951).

Goodman, J. R., W. H. Florsheim, and C. E. Tempereau: *Reserpine and thyroid function.* Proc. Soc. exp. Biol. Med. 90, 196—198 (1955).

Goodman, L. S., J. E. P. Toman, and E. A. Swinyard: *The anticonvulsant properties of tridione.* Amer. J. Med. 1, 213—228 (1946).

Govier, W. H., B. G. Homes, and A. J. Gibbons: *The oxidative deamination of serotonin and other 3-(beta-aminoethyl)-indoles by monoamine oxidase and the effect of the compounds on the deamination of tyramine.* Science 118, 596—597 (1963).

Gowdey, C. W., A. R. McKay, and D. Torney: *Effects of levomepromazine and chlorpromazine on conditioning and other responses of the nervous system.* Arch. int. Pharmacodyn. 123, 352—361 (1959).

Graham, R. C. B., F. C. Lu, and M. C. Allmark: *Combined effect of tranquilizing drugs and alcohol on rats.* Fed. Proc. 16, 302 (1957).

Green, H., and R. W. Erickson: *Effect of trans-2-phenyl-cyclopropylamine upon norepinephrine concentration and monoamine oxidase activity of rat brain.* J. Pharmacol. exp. Ther. 129, 237—242 (1960).

Green, H., and J. L. Sawyer: *Intracellular distribution of norepinephrine in rat brain. Effect of reserpine and the monoamine oxidase inhibitors, trans-2-phenylcyclopropylamine and 1-isonicotinyl-2-isopropyl hydrazine.* J. Pharmacol. exp. Ther. 129, 243—249 (1960).

Greig, M. E., R. A. Walk, and A. J. Gibbons: *The effect of three tryptamine derivatives on serotonin metabolism in vitro and in vivo.* J. Pharmacol. exp. Ther. 127, 110—115 (1959).

Greig, M. E., P. H. Slay, and W. A. Freiburger: The pharmacology of tryptamine. J. Neuropsychiatrie 2, 131—135 (1961).

Grenell, R. G., J. Mendelson, and W. D. McElroy: *Effects of chlorpromazine on metabolism in central nervous system.* Arch. Neurol. Psychiat. 73, 347—351 (1955).

Griesemer, E. G., C. A. Dragstedt, J. A. Wells, and E. A. Zeller: *Adrenergic blockade by iproniazid.* Experientia 11, 182—183 (1955).

Gros, H., M. Peterfalvi et R. Jequier: *Explorations à toutes doses d'un dérivé nonsédative de la réserpine, le R-694, dans le traitement de l'hypertension arterielle.* Algérie méd. 63, 297—298 (1959).

Gross, M., I. L. Hitchman, W. P. Reeves, J. Lawrence, and P. C. Newell: *Discontinuation of treatment with ataractic drugs.* In: Recent advances in biological psychiatry, Vol. III. Ed. J. Wortis. New York: Grune and Stratton, Inc. 1961, pp. 44—67.

Grünthal, E., u. H. Walther-Büel: *Über Schädigung der Oliva inferior durch Chlorperphenazin (Trilafon).* Psychiat. Neurol. (Basel) 140, 249—257 (1960).

Guerrero-Figueroa, R., and D. M. Gallant: *Effects of pinoxepin and imipramine on the mesencephalic reticular formation and amygdaloid complex in the cat: Neurophysiological and clinical correlations in human subjects.* Curr. Ther. Res. 9 (7), 387—403 (1967).

Gylys, J. A., P. M. R. Muccia, and M. K. Taylor: *Pharmacological and toxicological properties of 2-methyl-3-piperidinopyrazine, a new antidepressant.* Ann. N. Y. Acad. Sci. 107, 899—912 (1963).

Haase, H. J.: *Psychiatrische Erfahrungen mit Megaphen (Largactil) und dem Rauwolfiaalkaloid Serpasil unter dem Gesichtspunkt des psychomotorischen Parkinsonsyndroms.* Nervenarzt 26, 507—510 (1955).

—, and P. A. J. Janssen: *The action of neuroleptic drugs.* Amsterdam: North Holland Publ. Co. 1965.

Haefely, W., A. Hurlimann, and H. Thoenen: *Scheinbar paradoxe Beeinflussung von peripheren Noradrenalin-Wirkungen durch einige Thymoleptica.* Helv. Physiol. Pharmacol. Acta 22, 15—33 (1964).

Häfliger, F., and V. Burckhardt: *Iminodibenzyl- and related compounds.* Psychopharmacol. Agents 1, 35—101 (1964).

Hafkenschiel, J. H., A. M. Sellers, G. A. King, and M. W. Thorner: *Preliminary observation of the effects of parenteral reserpine on cerebral blood flow, oxygen and glucose metabolism, and EEG of patients with essential hypertension.* Ann. N. Y. Acad. Sci. 61, 78—84 (1955).

Hagen, P., and R. J. Barnett: *The storage of amines in the chromaffin cell.* In: Adrenergic mechanisms. Eds. J. R. Vane, G. E. W. Wolstenholme, and J. O'Connor. London: J. & A. Churchill, Ltd. 1960, pp. 83—99.

Haley, T. J., A. M. Flesher, and K. Raymond: *Pharmacological comparison of chlorpromazine and Mellaril, 3-methyl-mercapto-10-[2-(N-Methyl-2-piperdyl)-ethyl]-phenothiazine hydrochloride.* Arch. int. Pharmacodyn. 124, 455—460 (1960).

133

Halliwell, G., R. M. Quinton, and F. E. Williams: *A comparison of imipramine, chlorpromazine and related drugs in various tests involving autonomic functions and antagonism of reserpine.* Brit. J. Pharmacol. 23, 330—350 (1964).

Hamberger, B., and D. Masuoka: *Localization of catecholamine uptake in rat brain slices.* Acta pharmacol. (Kobenhaven) 22, 363—368 (1965).

Hamel, E. G., Jr., and W. W. Kaelber: *Reserpine action on the central nervous system of the cat.* Amer. J. Physiol. 200, 195—200 (1961).

Hammer, W., and F. Sjöqvist: *Inhibition of the metabolism of tremorine and oxotremorine in rats by antidepressants of the imipramine-type.* In: Antidepressant drugs. Eds. S. Garattini and M. N. G. Dukes. Amsterdam: Excerpta Medica Fdn. 1967, pp. 279—289.

Hanson, H. M., J. J. Witoslawski, E. H. Campbell, and A. G. Itkin: *Estimation of relative antiavoidance activity of depressant drugs in squirrel monkeys.* Arch. int. Pharmacodyn. 161 (1), 7—16 (1966).

Haot, J., B. Djahanguiri et M. Richelle: *Action protectrice du chlordiazepoxide sur l'ulcère de contrainte chez le rat.* Arch. int. Pharmacodyn. 148, 557—559 (1964).

Hardisty, R. M., G. I. C. Ingram, and R. S. Stacey: *Reserpine and human platelet 5-hydroxytryptamine.* Experientia 12, 424—425 (1956).

Harrer, G.: *Zur Inkompatibilität zwischen Monoaminoxydase-Hemmern und Imipramin.* Wien. med. Wschr. 111, 551—553 (1961).

Harwood, C. T., and J. W. Mason: *Acute effects of tranquilizing drugs on the anterior pituitary-ACTH mechanism.* Endocrinology 60, 239—246 (1957).

Hassler, R.: *Extrapyramidal-motorische Syndrome und Erkrankungen.* In: Hb. Inn. Med. Vol. III. Berlin-Göttingen-Heidelberg: Springer 1953, pp. 676—904.

Haverback, B. J., and D. F. Bodganski: *Gastric mucosal erosion in the rat following administration of the serotonin precursor, 5-hydroxytryptophan.* Proc. Soc. exp. Biol. Med. 95, 392—393 (1957).

Heimann, H., u. P. N. Witt: *Die Wirkung einer einmaligen Largactilgabe bei Gesunden.* Mschr. Psychiat. Neurol. 129, 104—128 (1955).

Heise, G. A., and E. Boff: *Behavioral determination of time and dose parameters of monoamine oxidase inhibitors.* J. Pharmacol. exp. Ther. 129, 155—162 (1960).

— — *Continuous avoidance as a base-line for measuring behavioral effects of drugs.* Psychopharmacologia 3, 264—282 (1962).

Helper, E. W., M. J. Carver, H. P. Jacobi, and J. A. Smith: *The effect of tranquilizing agents and related compounds on the succinoxidase systems.* Arch. Biochem. 76, 354—361 (1958).

Henatch, H. D., u. D. H. Ingvar: *Chlorpromazin und Spastizität: Eine elektrophysiologische Untersuchung.* Arch. Psychiat. 195, 77—93 (1956).

Hendley, C. D., T. E. Lynes, and F. M. Berger: *Effect of 2-methyl, 2-n-propyl-1, 3-propanediol dicarbamate (Miltown) on central nervous system.* Proc. Soc. exp. Biol. Med. 87, 608—610 (1954).

Hernandez-Peon, R., J. A. Rojas-Ramirez, J. J. O'Flaherty, and A. L. Mazzuchelli-O'Flaherty: *An experimental study of the anticonvulsive and relaxant actions of Valium.* Int. J. Neuropharmacol. 3, 405—412 (1964).

Herr, F., J. Stewart, and M.-P. Charest: *Tranquilizers and antidepressants: A pharmacological comparison.* Arch. int. Pharmacodyn. 134, 328—342 (1961).

Herrmann, B., W. Schindler, and R. Pulver: *Paper chromatographic determination of metabolic products of Tofranil.* Med. Exp. 1, 381—385 (1959).

— *Quantitative Methoden zur Untersuchung des Stoffwechsels von Tofranil®.* Helv. Physiol. Pharmacol. Acta 21, 402—408 (1963).

Hertting, G., u. O. Hornykiewicz: *Beeinflussung der durch Reserpin hervorgerufenen Nebennierenrindenhypertrophie durch Cortison.* Acta endocrinol. 26, 204 bis 208 (1957).

Hertting, G.: *Über den Einfluß des Serotoninstoffwechsels auf die Metrazolkrampf-schwelle bei Mäusen.* Wien. klin. Wschr. 70, 190—192 (1958).

—, u. E. Stoklaska: *Über den Einfluß nervöser Faktoren auf das Dextranödem der Rattenpfote und auf die ödemhemmende Wirkung von Chlorpromazin.* Naunyn-Schmiedeberg Arch. exp. Path. 237, 423—429 (1959).

—, and J. Axelrod: *Fate of tritiated noradrenaline at the sympathetic nerve endings.* Nature 192, 172—173 (1961).

— —, and L. G. Whitby: *Effect of drugs on the uptake and metabolism of H^3-norepinephrine.* J. Pharmacol. exp. Ther. 134, 146—153 (1961).

—, L. T. Potter, and J. Axelrod: *Effect of decentralization and ganglionic blocking agents on the spontaneous release of H^3-norepinephrine.* J. Pharmacol. exp. Ther. 136, 289—292 (1962).

Hess, S. M., B. G. Redfield, and S. Undenfriend: *The effect of monoamine oxidase inhibitors and tryptophane on the tryptamine content of animal tissues and urine.* J. Pharmacol. exp. Ther. 127, 178—181 (1959).

Hiebel, G., M. Bonvallet et P. Dell: *Action de la chlorpromazine ("largactil"), (4560 RP) au niveau du system nerveux central.* Sem. Hop. Paris, 30, 2346—2354 (1954).

Hillarp, N.-A., S. Lagerstedt, and B. Nilson: *The isolation of a granular fraction from the suprarenal medulla, containing the sympathomimetic catecholamines.* Acta Physiol. scand. 29, 251—263 (1953).

— *Effect of reserpine on the adrenal medulla of sheep.* Acta Physiol. scand. 49, 376—382 (1960 a).

— *Different pools of catecholamines stored in the adrenal medulla.* Acta Physiol. scand. 50, 8—22 (1960 b).

Himwich, H. E., F. Rinaldi, and D. Willis: *An examination of phenothiazine derivatives with comparisons of their effects on the alerting reaction, chemical structure and therapeutic efficacy.* J. nerv. ment. Dis. 124, 53—57 (1956).

—, and F. Rinaldi: *Analysis of the action of benzotropine methanesulfonate against parkinsonism.* In: Tranquilizing drugs. Amer. Ass. for the Advancement of Science. Publ. No. 46, pp. 47—57 (1957).

— *Experiments with alphamethyltryptamine.* J. Neuropsychiat. 2 (Suppl.), 136 to 140 (1961).

—, G. Brune, W. Steiner, and H. Kohl: *A pharmacological study of terminal methyl groups in animals.* Recent Advances Biol. Psychiat. 6, 196—207 (1964).

Himwich, W. A., and S. N. Glisson: *Effect of haloperidol on caudate nucleus.* Int. J. Neuropharmacol. 6, 329—332 (1967).

—, and J. C. Petersen: *Effect of the combined administration of imipramine and a monoamine oxidase inhibitor.* Amer. J. Psychiat. 117, 928—929 (1961).

Hirschmann, J., u. K. Mayer: *Zur Beeinflussung der Akinese und anderer extrapyramidalmotorischer Störungen mit L-DOPA (L-Dihydroxyphenylalanin).* Dtsch. med. Wschr. 89, 1877—1880 (1964).

Hollister, L. E.: *Complications from use of tranquilizing drugs.* New Engl. J. Med. 257, 170—177 (1957).

—, and F. S. Glazener: *Withdrawal reactions from meprobamate alone and combined with promazine—a control study.* Psychopharmacologia 1, 336—341 (1960).

—, F. P. Motzenbecker, and R. O. Degen: *Withdrawal reactions from chlordiazepoxide ("Librium").* Psychopharmacologia 2, 63—68 (1961).

— *Current concepts in therapy. Complications from psychotherapeutic drugs II.* New Engl. J. Med. 264, 345—347 (1961).

Hollister, L. E.: *Complications from psychotherapeutic drugs*-1964. Clin. Pharmacol. Ther. **5**, 322—333 (1964).

Holtz, P., H. Balzer u. E. Westermann: *Beeinflussung der Reserpinwirkung auf das Nebennierenmark durch Hemmung der Mono-aminoxydase*. Naunyn-Schmiedeberg Arch. exp. Path. **231**, 361—372 (1957 a).

— — — u. E. Wezler: *Beeinflussung der Evipannarkose durch Reserpin, Iproniazid und biogene Amine*. Naunyn-Schmiedeberg Arch. exp. Path. **231**, 333—348 (1957 b).

—, W. Osswald u. K. Stock: *Über die Beeinflussung der Wirkungen sympathikominetischer Amine durch Cocain und Reserpin*. Naunyn-Schmiedeberg Arch. exp. Path. **239**, 14—28 (1960).

Holzbauer, M., and M. Vogt: *The action of chlorpromazine on diencephalic sympathetic activity and on the release of adrenocorticotrophic hormone*. Brit. J. Pharmacol. **9**, 402—407 (1954).

— — *Depression by reserpine of the noradrenaline concentration in the hypothalamus of the cat*. J. Neurochem. **1**, 8—11 (1956).

Holzer, G., u. O. Hornykiewicz: *Über den Dopamin-(Hydroxytyramin-)Stoffwechsel im Gehirn der Ratte*. Naunyn-Schmiedeberg Arch. exp. Path. **237**, 27 bis 33 (1959).

Hooper, J. H., Jr., V. C. Welch, and R. T. Schackelford: *Abnormal lactation associated with tranquilizing drug therapy*. J. Amer. med. Ass. **178**, 506—507 (1961).

Horita, A.: *A vasopressor response to reserpine in the cocainized dog*. J. Pharmacol. exp. Ther. **122**, 474—479 (1958).

—, and W. R. McGrath: *The interaction between reversible and irreversible monoamine oxidase inhibitors*. Biochem. Pharmacol. **3**, 206—211 (1960).

—, and C. Chinn: *An analysis of the interaction of reversible and irreversible monoamine oxidase inhibitors*. Biochem. Pharmacol. **13**, 371—378 (1964).

Hornykiewicz, O., H. Ehringer u. K. Lechner: *Beeinflussung der Iproniazidwirkung auf die Katecholamine und das 5-Hydroxytryptamin des Rattenhirnes durch Chlorpromazin*. Naunyn-Schmiedeberg Arch. exp. Path. **241**, 198—199 (1961).

— *Die topische Lokalisation und das Verhalten von Noradrenalin und Dopamin (3-Hydroxytyramin) in der Substantia nigra des normalen und Parkinson-kranken Menschen*. Wien. klin. Wschr. **75**, 309—312 (1963).

— *Zur Existenz „dopaminerger" Neurone im Gehirn*. Naunyn-Schmiedeberg Arch. exp. Path. **247**, 304—305 (1964 a).

— *Zur Frage des Verlaufs dopaminerger Neurone im Gehirn des Menschen*. Wien. klin. Wschr. **76**, 834—835 (1964 b).

— *The role of brain dopamine (3-hydroxytyramine) in parkinsonism*. In: Biochemical and neurophysiological correlation of centrally acting drugs. Oxford-London-Edinburgh-New York-Paris-Frankfurt: Pergamon Press 1964 c, pp. 57 to 68.

— *Neuere Aspekte der biochemischen Pharmakologie des Parkinson-Syndroms*. Wien. Z. Nervenheilk. **23**, 103—109 (1966 a)

— *Dopamine (3-hydroxytyramine) and brain function*. Pharmacol. Rev. **18**, 925—964 (1966 b).

Horovitz, Z. P., A. R. Furgiuele, L. J. Brannick, J. C. Burke, and B. N. Craver: *A new chemical structure with specific depressant effects on the amygdala and on the hyper-irritability of the "septal rat"*. Nature **200**, 369—370 (1963).

—, P. W. Ragozzino, and R. C. Leaf: *Select block of rat mouse-killing by antidepressants*. Life Sci. **4**, 1909—1912 (1965).

Horwitz, D., L. I. Goldberg, and A. Sjoerdsma: *Possible hemodynamic basis for beneficial effects of a monoamine oxidase inhibitor in angina pectoris.* Circulation 24, 959—960 (1961).

Hucker, H. B.: *Metabolism of amitriptyline.* Pharmacologist 4, 171 (1962).

Hudson, R. D., and E. F. Domino: *Evidence for a brainstem action of chlorpromazine on some motor reflexes.* Fed. Proc. 20, 307 (1961).

Huebner, C. F., and E. Wenkert: *Rauwolfia alkaloids XXII. Further observations of the sterochemistry of reserpine.* J. Amer. Chem. Soc. 77, 4180 (1955).

—, H. B. McPhillamy, E. Schlittler, and A. F. St. Andre: *Rauwolfia alkaloids XXI. The sterochemistry of reserpine and deserpidine.* Experientia 11, 303—304 (1955).

Hughes, F. B., and B. B. Brodie: *The mechanism of serotonin and catecholamine uptake by platelets.* J. Pharmacol. exp. Ther. 127, 96—102 (1959).

Huidobro, F.: *Some pharmacological properties of chloro-3(dimethylamine-3'-propyl)10-phenothiazine or 4.560 R. P.* Arch. int. Pharmacodyn. 98, 308—319 (1954).

Huković, S., u. E. Muscholl: *Die Noradrenalinabgabe aus dem isolierten Kaninchenherzen bei sympathischer Nervenreizung und ihre pharmakologische Beeinflussung.* Naunyn-Schmiedeberg Arch. exp. Path. 244, 81—96 (1962).

Hunt, H.: *Some effects of meprobamate on conditioned fear and emotional behavior.* Ann. N. Y. Acad. Sci. 67, 712—723 (1957).

Hunter, R., C. J. Earl, and S. Thornicroft: *An apparently irreversible syndrome of abnormal movements following phenothiazine medication.* Proc. roy. Soc. Med. 57, 758—762 (1964).

Iggo, A., and M. Vogt: *Preganglionic sympathetic activity in normal and in reserpine-treated cats.* J. Physiol. 150, 114—133 (1960).

Innes, I. R., O. Krayer, and D. R. Wand: *The action of rauwolfia alkaloids on the heart rate and on the functional refractory period of atrio-ventricular transmission in the heart-lung preparation of the dog.* J. Pharmacol. exp. Ther. 124, 324—332 (1958).

Inouye, A., and I. Tanaka: *Effect of tyramine, reserpine and cocaine on the noradrenaline release and uptake of the perfused rabbit kidney.* Acta physiol. scand. 62, 359—363 (1964).

Isaac, L., and A. Goth: *Interaction of antihistaminics with norepinephrine uptake: a cocaine-like effect.* Life Sci. 4, 1899—1904 (1965).

Jacobsen, E.: *The comparative pharmacology of some psychotropic drugs.* Bull. WHO 21, 411—493 (1959).

Janssen, P. A. J.: *Comparative pharmacological data on 6 new basic 4'-fluoro-butyrophenone derivatives: haloperidol, haloanisone, Triperidol®, methylperidide, haloperidide and dipiperone.* Arzneimittel-Forsch. (Ger.) 11, 819—824 (1961).

— *The pharmacology of haloperiod.* Int. J. Neuropsychiat. 3 (S 1), S 10—S 18 (1967).

—, and C. J. E. Niemegeers: *Chemistry and pharmacology of compounds related to 4-(4-hydroxy-4-phenyl-piperidino)-butyrophenone.* Arzneimittel-Forsch. 9, 765—767 (1959).

—, A. J. Jageneau, and C. J. E. Niemegeers: *Effects of various isolation-induced fighting behavior of male mice.* J. Pharmacol. exp. Ther. 129, 471—475 (1960).

—, C. J. E. Niemegeers, and K. H. L. Schellekens: *Is it possible to predict the clinical effects of neuroleptic drugs (major tranquilizers) from animal data? Part II. "Neuroleptic activity spectra" for dogs.* Arzneimittel-Forsch. 15, 1196 (1965).

Jaramillo, G. A. V. de, and P. S. Guth: *A study of the localization of pheno-thiazines in dog brain*. Biochem. Pharmacol. 12, 525—532 (1963).

Jenney, E. H.: *Changes in convulsant thresholds after rauwolfia serpentina, reserpine and veriloid*. Fed. Proc. 13, 370—371 (1954).

Jiménez-Pabón, E., and R. A. Nelson: *Quantitative measurements of muscle tone in cats*. Neurology 15, 1120—1126 (1965).

Jindal, M. N., and V. R. Deshpande: *Neuromuscular blockade by some pheno-thiazine derivatives*. Arch. int. Pharmacodyn. 132, 322—330 (1961).

Jori, A., and S. Garattini: *Interaction between imipramine-like agents and catecholamine-induced hyperthermia*. J. Pharm. Pharmacol. 17, 480—488 (1965).

—, S. Paglialunga, and S. Garattini: *Adrenergic mediation in the antagonism between desipramine and reserpine*. J. Pharm. Pharmacol. 18, 326—327 (1966).

Jourdan, F., P. Duchêne-Marullaz et P. Boissier: *Étude expérimentale de l'action de la chlorpromazine sur les système nerveux végétatif*. Arch. int. Pharmacodyn. 101, 253—278 (1955).

Julon, L., O. Leau, R. Ducrot, J. Fournel et M. C. Bardone: *Propriété pharmaco-dynamique général du (diméthylamino-3'-méthyl-2'-propyl-1')-5-iminodibenzyle (7.162 R. P.) et de ses isomeres optiques, droit (10.633) R. P.) et gauche (10.645 R. P.)*. C. R. Soc. Biol. 155, 307—312 (1961).

Kakimoto, Y., and M. D. Armstrong: *On the identification of octopamine in mammals*. J. Biol. Chem. 237, 422—427 (1962).

Kalow, W.: *Pharmacogenetics*. Philadelphia—London. W. B. Saunders Co. 1962.

Karki, N. T., M. K. Paasonen, and P. A. Vanhakartano: *The influence of pentolonium, isoraunescine and yohimbine on the noradrenaline depleting action of reserpine*. Acta Pharmacol. 16, 13—19 (1959).

Kato, R., E. Chiesara, and P. Vassanelli: *Mechanism of potentiation of barbiturates and meprobamate actions by imipramine*. Biochem. Pharmacol. 12, 357—364 (1963).

Kaumann, A. J., and N. Basso: *Inhibitory action of desmethylimipramine on the restoration of the pressor effect of tyramine and on the uptake of noradrenaline in the reserpinized dog*. Arch. int. Pharmacodyn. 160 (1), 113—123 (1966).

Khan, A. U., R. B. Forney, and F. W. Hughes: *Plasma free fatty acids in rats after shock as modified by centrally active drugs*. Arch. int. Pharmacodyn. 151, 466—474 (1964).

Khazan, N., F. G. Sulman, and H. Z. Winnik: *Effect of reserpine on pituitary-gonadal axis*. Proc. Soc. exp. Biol. Med. 105, 201—204 (1960).

Kido, R., and K. Yamamoto: *A comparative analysis of behavioral and electro-encephalographic changes caused by CNS depressants in animal experiments*. Neuropsychopharmacology 4, 327—333 (1965).

Kielholz, P. (Hrsg.): *Psychiatrische Pharmakotherapie in Klinik und Praxis*. Bern—Stuttgart: Hans Huber 1965.

Kikuchi, T.: *Electroencephalographic studies on the action of reserpine in the rabbit and combined action of reserpine and methamphetamine*. Folia Pharmacol. Jap. 57, 173—192 (1961).

Killam, E. K., and K. F. Killam: *A comparison of the effects of reserpine and chlorpromazine to those of barbiturates on central afferent systems in the cat*. J. Pharmacol. exp. Ther. 116, 35 (1956).

— — *The influence of drugs on central afferent pathways*. In: Brain mechanisms and drug action. Ed. W. Fields, pp. 71—94. Springfield, Ill.: C. C. Thomas 1957.

— —, and T. Shaw: *The effects of psychotherapeutic compounds on central afferent and limbic pathways*. Ann. N. Y. Acad. Sci. 66, 784—805 (1957).

Killam, E. K., and K. F. Killam: *Phenothiazine-pharmacologic studies.* Ass. Res. nerv. Dis. Proc. 37, 245—265 (1959).
— *Drug action on the brain-stem reticular formation.* Pharmacol. Rev. 14, 175 to 223 (1962).
Killam, K. F.: *Pharmacological influences upon evoked electrical activity in the brain.* In: Psychotropic drugs. Eds. S. Garattini and V. Ghetti. Amsterdam: Elsevier Publ. Co. 1957, pp. 244—251.
Kim, K. S., and P. A. Shore: *Mechanism of action of reserpine and insulin on gastric amines and gastric acid secretion, and the effect of monoamine oxidase inhibition.* J. Pharmacol. exp. Ther. 141, 321—325 (1963).
Kirpekar, S. M., G. A. J. Goodlad, and J. J. Lewis: *Reserpine depletion of adenosine triphosphate from the rat suprarenal medulla.* Biochem. Pharmacol. 1, 232—233 (1958).
—, and J. J. Lewis: *Some effects of reserpine and hydralazine upon tissue respiration and the concentration of adenosine nucleotides in certain tissues.* Brit. J. Pharmacol. 14, 40—45 (1959).
Kirshner, N.: *Pathway of noradrenaline formation from DOPA.* J. Biol. Chem. 226, 821—825 (1957).
— *Uptake of catecholamines by a particulate fraction of the adrenal medulla.* Science 135, 107—108 (1962 a).
— *Uptake of catecholamines by a particulate fraction of the adrenal medulla.* J. Biol. Chem. 237, 2311—2317 (1962 b).
—, M. Robie, and D. L. Kamin: *Inhibition of dopamine uptake in vitro by reserpine administered in vivo.* J. Pharmacol. exp. Ther. 141, 285—289 (1963).
Kitay, J. L., D. A. Holub, and J. W. Jailer: *"Inhibition" of pituitary ACTH release after administration of reserpine or epinephrine.* Endocrinology 65, 548—554 (1959).
Kletzkin, M., and F. M. Berger: *Effect of meprobamate on limbic system of the brain.* Proc. Soc. exp. Biol. Med. 100, 681—683 (1959).
—, and K. Swan: *The effects of meprobamate and pentobarbital upon cortical and subcortical responses to auditory stimulation.* J. Pharmacol. exp. Ther. 125, 35—39 (1959).
Klupp, H., and J. Kahling: *Pharmakologische Wirkungen von 7-Chlor-1,3-dihydro-3-hydroxy-5-phenyl-2H-1,4-Benzodiazepin-2-on.* Arzneimittel-Forsch. 15, 359—365 (1965).
Kobinger, W.: *Differentiation between the sedative actions of 5-hydroxytryptamine and reserpine in mice by means of two stimulating substances.* Acta Pharmacol. 14, 138—147 (1958 a).
— *Reversibility of a facilitatory action of reserpine on the central nervous system by methylamphetamine.* Experientia 14, 337—338 (1958 b).
Koechlin, B. A., M. A. Schwartz, G. Krol, and W. Oberhansli: *The metabolic fate of C^{14}-labeled chlordiazepoxide in man, in the dog, and in the rat.* J. Pharmacol. exp. Ther. 148, 399—411 (1965).
Konzett, H.: *Förderung von Schlaf und Narkose durch Farbstoffe.* Naunyn-Schmiedeberg Arch. exp. Path. 188, 349—359 (1938).
Kopera, J., and A. K. Armitage: *Comparison of some pharmacological properties of chlorpromazine, promethazine, and pethidine.* Brit. J. Pharmacol. 9, 392 to 401 (1954).
Kopin, I. J., and J. Axelrod: *The metabolic fate of epinephrine in the rat.* Fed. Proc. 19, 295 (1960).
—, and E. K. Gordon: *Metabolism of norepinephrine-H^3 released by tyramine and reserpine.* J. Pharmacol. exp. Ther. 138, 351—359 (1962).

Kopin, I. J., and E. K. Gordon: *Metabolism of administered and drug-released norepinephrine-7-H³ in the rat.* J. Pharmacol. exp. Ther. 140, 207—216 (1963).

—, G. Hertting, and E. K. Gordon: *Fate of norepinephrine-H³ in the isolated perfused rat heart.* J. Pharmacol. exp. Ther. 138, 34—40 (1962).

— *Storage and metabolism of catecholamines: The role of monoamine oxidase.* Pharmacol. Rev. 16, 179—191 (1964).

—, J. E. Fischer, J. Musacchio, and W. D. Horst: *Evidence for a false neurochemical transmitter as a mechanism for the hypotensive effect of monoamine oxidase inhibitors.* Proc. nat. Acad. Sci. (Wash.) 52, 716—721 (1964).

Kornetsky, C., and O. Humphries: *Psychological effects of centrally acting drugs in man. Effects of chlorpromazine and secobarbital and visual and motor behavior.* J. ment. Sci. 104, 1093—1099 (1958).

— *Alterations in psychomotor functions and individual differences in responses produced by psychoactive drugs.* In: Drugs and behavior. Eds. L. Uhr and J. G. Miller. New York: John Wiley & Sons, Inc. 1960, pp. 297—312.

Kouzmanoff, S. P., D. K. Eckfeld, R. Tislow, and J. Seifter: *Meprobamate and phenothiazine antagonism to some morphine-induced phenomena in the mouse.* J. Pharmacol. exp. Ther. 22, 40 A (1958).

Krayer, O., and J. Fuentes: *Changes of heart rate caused by direct cardiac action of reserpine.* J. Pharmacol. exp. Ther. 123, 145—152 (1958).

Krivoy, W. A.: *Actions of chlorpromazine and of reserpine on spinal reflex activity in the cat.* Proc. Soc. exp. Biol. Med. 96, 18—20 (1957).

Kroneberg, G., u. H. J. Schümann: *Die Wirkung des Reserpins auf den Hormongehalt des Nebennierenmarks.* Naunyn-Schmiedeberg Arch. exp. Path. 231, 349 bis 360 (1957).

— — *Adrenalinsekretion und Adrenalinverarmung der Kaninchennebennieren nach Reserpin.* Naunyn-Schmiedeberg Arch. exp. Path. 234, 133—146 (1958).

Kuhn, R.: *Über die Behandlung depressiver Zustände mit einem Iminodibenzylderivat (G-22355).* Schweiz. med. Wschr. 87, 1135—1140 (1957).

Kuntzman, R., S. Udenfriend, E. G. Tomich, B. B. Brodie, and P. A. Shore: *Biochemical effects of reserpine on serotonin binding sites.* Fed. Proc. 15, 450 (1956).

Kuschinsky, G., R. Lindmar, H. Lullmann u. E. Muscholl: *Der Einfluß von Reserpin auf die Wirkung der „Neurosympathikomimetica".* Naunyn-Schmiedeberg Arch. exp. Path. 240, 242—252 (1960).

Kuschke, H. J.: u. H. V. Ditrurth: *Die Ausscheidung von Noradrenalin und Adrenalin unter hochdosierter Reserpinbehandlung.* Klin. Wschr. 36, 773—774 (1958).

—, u. J. Frantz: *Über eine hyperglykämische Wirkung von Reserpin.* Naunyn-Schmiedeberg Arch. exp. Path. 224, 269—274 (1955).

Laborit, H., et P. Huguenard: *L'hibernation artificielle par moyens pharmacodynamiques et physiques.* Presse méd. 59, 1329 (1951).

— — *Technique actuelle de l'hibernation artificielle.* Presse méd. 60, 1455—1456 (1952).

Labrosse, E. H., and G. Hertting: *Biliary excretion of DL-epinephrine metabolites.* Fed. Proc. 19, 297 (1960).

Lanoir, J., G. Dolce, and E. Chirinos: *Étude neurophysiologique du RO 4-5360.* C. R. Soc. Biol. (Paris) 159, 431—435 (1965).

Lapin, I. P.: *Comparison of antireserpine and anticholinergic effects of antidepressants and of central and peripheral cholinolytics.* In: Antidepressant drugs. Eds. S. Garattini and M. N. G. Dukes. Amsterdam: Excerpta Medica Fdn. 1967, pp. 266—278.

Laroche, M. J., and B. B. Brodie: *Lack of relationship between inhibition of monoamine oxidase and potentiation of hexobarbital hypnosis.* J. Pharmacol. exp. Ther. **130**, 134—137 (1960).

Lasagna, L., and W. P. MacCann: *Aggregation, amphetamine and "tranquilizers".* Fed. Proc. **16**, 315 (1957).

Laverty, R., and D. F. Sharman: *Modification by drugs of the metabolism of 3,4-dihydroxyphenylethylamine, noradrenaline and 5-hydroxytryptamine in the brain.* Brit. J. Pharmacol. **24**, 759—772 (1965).

Lee, W. C., Y. H. Shin, and F. E. Shideman: *Cardiac activities of several monoamine oxidase inhibitors.* J. Pharmacol. exp. Ther. **133**, 180—185 (1961).

Lehmann, H. E., and J. Csank: *Differential screening of phrenotropic agents in man: Psychophysiologic test data.* J. Clin. exp. Psychopath. **18**, 222—235 (1957).

—, and T. A. Ban (eds.): *The Butyrophenones in psychiatry. First North American Symposium on the Butyrophenones.* Quebec Psychopharmacological Research Association, 1964.

Lembeck, F.: *5-Hydroxytryptamine in carcinoid tumor.* Nature **172**, 910—911 (1953).

Le Roy, J. G., and A. F. de Schaepdryver: *Catecholamine levels of brain and heart in mice after iproniazid, syrosingopine and 10-methoxydeserpidine.* Arch. int. Pharmacodyn. **130**, 231—234 (1961).

Leslie, G. B., and D. R. Maxwell: *Some pharmacological properties of thioproperazine and their modification by anti-parkinsonian drugs.* Brit. J. Pharmacol. **22**, 301—317 (1964).

Lewis, J. J.: *Rauwolfia derivatives.* In: Physiological Pharmacology, Vol. I, Part A. Eds. W. S. Root and F. G. Hofmann. New York-London: Academic Press 1963, pp. 479—536.

Liebman, H., and H. Matthies: *Der Einfluß des Reserpins auf die Toxizität cholinerger Pharmaka.* Acta biol. med. germ. **13**, 586—590 (1964).

Lindmar, R., u. E. Muscholl: *Die Wirkung von Cocain, Guanethidin, Reserpin, Hexamethonium, Tetracain und Psicain auf die Noradrenalin-Freisetzung aus dem Herzen.* Naunyn-Schmiedeberg Arch. exp. Path. **242**, 214—227 (1961).

— — *Die Wirkung von Pharmaka auf die Elimination von Noradrenalin aus der Perfusionsflüssigkeit und die Noradrenalinaufnahme in das isolierte Herz.* Naunyn-Schmiedeberg Arch. exp. Path. **247**, 469—492 (1964).

Lisovskaya, N. P., and N. B. Livanova: Cit. J. J. Lewis.

Loew, D.: *Untersuchungen über die aminpotenzierenden Wirkungen von antidepressiv wirkenden Stoffen am Kaninchen.* Med. exp. **11**, 333—351 (1964).

—, and M. Taeschler: *Central anticholinergic properties of antidepressants.* In: Neuropsychopharmacology, Vol. IV. Eds. D. Bente and B. P. Bradley. Amsterdam: Elsevier Publ. Co. 1965, pp. 404—407.

Löw, H.: *On the participation of flavin in mitochondrial adenosine triphosphatase reactions.* Biochem. Biophys. Acta **32**, 1—20 (1959).

Loewe, S.: *Influence of chlorpromazine, reserpine, dibenzyline and desoxycorticosterone upon morphine-induced feline mania.* Arch. int. Pharmacodyn. **108**, 453—456 (1956).

Longo, V. G., G. P. von Berger, and D. Bovet: *Action of nicotine and of the "ganglioplegiques centraux" on the electrical activity of the rabbit brain.* J. Pharmacol. exp. Ther. **111**, 349—359 (1954).

— *Action de la chlorpromazine, de la lévomepromazine et de la prochlorpérazine sur l'activité électrique cérébral et sur le comportement du lapin.* Electroenceph. clin. Neurophysiol. **12**, 693—704 (1960).

Loomer, H. P., J. C. Saunders, and N. S. Kline: *A clinical and pharmacodynamic evaluation of iproniazid as a psychic energizer.* Psychiat. Res. Rep. Amer. psychiat. Ass. 8, 129 (1957).

MacLean, P. D., S. Flanigan, J. P. Flynn, C. Fim, and J. R. Stevens: *Hippocampal function; tentative correlations of conditioning, EEG, drug and radioautographic studies.* Yale J. Biol. Med. 28, 380—395 (1955—1956).

Mafouz, M., and E. A. Ezz: *The effect of reserpine and chlorpromazine on the response of the rat to acute stress.* J. Pharmacol. exp. Ther. 123, 39—42 (1958).

Maling, H. M., B. Highman, and S. Spector: *Neurologic, neuropathologic, and neurochemical effects of prolonged administration of phenylisopropylhydrazine (JB 516), phenylisobutylhydrazine (JB 835) and other monoamine oxidase inhibitors.* J. Pharmacol. exp. Ther. 137, 334—343 (1962).

Malmfors, R.: *Studies on adrenergic nerves.* Acta Physiol. scand. 64 (Supp. 248), 1—93 (1965).

Malthora, C. L., and R. K. Sidhu: *Anti-emetic activity of alkaloids of rauwolfia serpentina.* J. Pharmacol. exp. Ther. 116, 123—129 (1956).

Manara, L., M. G. Sestini, S. Algeri, and S. Garattini: *On the ability of des-imipramine to interfere with reserpine-induced noradrenaline release.* J. Pharm. Pharmacol. 18, 194—195 (1966).

Margules, D. L., and L. Stein: *Neuroleptics vs Tranquilizers: Evidence from animal behavior studies of mode and site of action.* In: Neuropsychopharmacology, Proc. of the Fifth International Congress, Washington, D. C. Eds. H. Brill et al. Amsterdam: Excerpta Medica Fdn. 1967, pp. 108—120.

Marrazzi, A. S.: *The effects of certain drugs on cerebral synapses.* Ann. N. Y. Acad. Sci. 66, 496—507 (1957).

Marriott, A. S., and P. S. Spencer: *Effects of centrally acting drugs on exploratory behavior in rats.* Brit. J. Pharmacol. 25, 432—441 (1965).

Martin, W. R., E. W. J. De Maar, and K. R. Unna: *Chlorpromazine, I. The action of chlorpromazine and related phenothiazines on the EEG and its activation.* J. Pharmacol. exp. Ther. 122, 343—358 (1958).

—, J. L. Riehl, and K. R. Unna: *Chlorpromazine, III. The effects of chlorpromazine and chlorpromazine sulfoxide on vascular responses to L-epinephrine and levarterenol.* J. Pharmacol. exp. Ther. 130, 37—45 (1960).

Masak, S., J. Metyš, and Z. Votava: *Antagonism of benactyzine, trihexphenidyl and three antidepressants against arecoline and tremorine-induced "analgesia", tremor and discoordination in mice.* Activ. nerv. Sup. 7, 282 (1965).

Matsuoka, M., H. Yoshida, and R. Imaizumi: *Correlation between brain catechol-amine and sedative action of reserpine.* Nature 202, 198 (1964).

Matthews, R. J., B. J. Roberts, and P. K. Adkins: *Neuropharmacological studies on dl-alphaethyltryptamine acetate.* J. Neuropsychiat. 2 (S), 151—158 (1961).

Matussek, N, u. U. Patschke: *Beziehungen des Schlaf- und Wachrhythmus zum Noradrenalin- und Serotoningehalt im Zentralnervensystem von Hamstern.* Med. exp. 11, 81—87 (1964).

—, E. Rüther, and E. O. Titus: *Einfluß und Wirkungsmechanismus adrenalin-potenzierender Pharmaka auf die Reserpinsedation.* Arzneimittelforschung 14, 503—505 (1964).

Maxwell, R. A., A. J. Plummer, S. D. Ross, and M. W. Osborne: *Effects of reser-pine on urinary bladder tension.* Proc. Soc. exp. Biol. Med. 92, 227—230 (1965).

—, S. D. Ross, A. J. Plummer, E. B. Sigg: *A peripheral action of reserpine.* J. Pharmacol. exp. Ther. 119, 69—77 (1957).

Mayer, S. W., F. H. Kelly, and M. E. Morton: *The direct antithyroid action of reserpine, chlorpromazine and other drugs.* J. Pharmacol. exp. Ther. 117, 197—201 (1956).

Maynert, E. W.: *Metabolic fate of drugs.* Ann Rev. Pharmacol. 1, 45—64 (1961).

McIlwain, H., and O. Greengard: *Excitants and depressants of the central nervous system, on isolated electrically-stimulated cerebral tissues.* J. Neurochem. 1, 348—357 (1957).

McQueen, E. G.: cit. H. J. Bein (1956).

McQuillen, M. P., M. Gross, and R. J. Jones: *Chlorpromazine-induced weakness in myasthenia gravis.* Arch. Neurol. 8, 286—290 (1963).

Meidinger, F.: *Action comparée des produits nos. 3.277 R. P., 4.560 R. P., 4.909 R. P. et du phénobarbital sur les convulsions provoquées par la strychnine, la picrotoxine, la cocaine, la caffeine et l'amphetamine.* C. R. Soc. Biol. (Paris) 150, 1340—1343 (1956).

Meier, R., C. Brüni et J. Tripod: *Différenciation pharmacodynamique de l'aprésoline, du serpasil et de la chlorpromazine lors de leur action sur la rétention hydrique du rat.* Arch. int. Pharmacodyn. 104, 137—145 (1955).

Mercier, J., P. Etzensperger, and S. Dessaigue: *Essai de localisation et d'interprétation de l'action de l'amitryptyline au niveau du système nerveux.* J. Physiol. 55, 581—609 (1963).

Metys, J., and J. Metysova: *Relationships between antrireserpine and central cholinolytic effects of imipramine-like antidepressants.* In: Antidepressant drugs. Eds. S. Garattini and M. N. G. Dukes. Amsterdam: Excerpta Medica Fdn. 1967, pp. 255—265.

Metyšová, J., J. Metyš, and Z. Votava: *Pharmakologische Eigenschaften einiger neuer Tranquiliziers und antidepressiven Substanzen.* Arch. int. Pharmacodyn. 144, 481—513 (1963).

Miline, R., P. Stern, E. Serstney et M. Muhibic: *Effect de la réserpine et de la resérpine associée au luminal sur le complexe hypothalamohypophysaire.* In: Psychotrop. drugs. Eds. S. Garattini and V. Ghetti. Amsterdam: Elsevier Publ. Co., 1957, pp. 332—349.

Mirkin, B. L.: *Catecholamine depletion in the rat's denervated adrenal gland following chronic administration of reserpine.* Nature 182, 113—114 (1958).

Mitoma, C., H. S. Posner, D. F. Bogdanski, and S. Udenfriend: *Biochemical and pharmacological studies on o-tyrosine and its meta and para analogues. A suggestion concerning phenylketonuria.* J. Pharmacol. exp. Ther. 120, 188—194 (1957).

Møller Nielsen, I., and K. Neuhold: *The comparative pharmacology and toxicity of the trans-isomer of 2-chloro-9-(3'-dimethylamino-propyledene)-thiaxanthene, HCL (Chlorprothixene)=N 714 trans anal chlorpromazine.* Acta Pharmacol. 15, 335—355 (1959).

—, W. Hougs, N. Lassen, T. Holm, and P. V. Petersen: *Central depressant activity of some thiaxanthene derivatives.* Acta Pharmacol. 19, 87—100 (1962).

Mörsdorf, K., and H. H. Bode: *Zur Beeinflussung der permeabilitäts-steigernden Wirkung des Serotonins durch verschiedenartige Pharmaka.* Arch. int. Pharmacodyn. 118, 292—297 (1959).

Monnier, M., u. P. Krupp: *Elektrophysiologische Analyse der Wirkungen verschiedener Neuroleptika (Chlorpromazine, Reserpin, Tofranil, Meprobamat).* Schweiz. med. Wschr. 89, 430—433 (1959).

—, et S. Graber: *Classification électrophysiologique des substances psycholeptiques (Position du chlordiazepoxide "Librium").* Arch. int. Pharmacodyn. 140, 206—216 (1962).

Monroe, R. R., R. G. Heath, W. A. Mickle, and W. Miller: *A comparison of cortical and subcortical brain waves in normal, barbiturate, reserpine and chlorpromazine sleep.* Ann. N. Y. Acad. Sci. 61, 56—71 (1955).

Montagu, K. A.: *Catechol compounds in rat tissues and in brains of different animals.* Nature 180, 244—245 (1957).

Moon, R. C., and C. W. Turner: *A mode of action for thyroid inhibition by reserpine*. Proc. Soc. exp. Biol. Med. **102**, 134—136 (1959).

Moore, J. I., and N. C. Moran: *Cardiac contractile force responses to ephedrine and other sympathomimetic amines in dogs after pretreatment with reserpine*. J. Pharmacol. exp. Ther. **136**, 89—96 (1962).

Moran, N. C., and W. M. Butler, Jr.: *The pharmacological properties of chlorpromazine sulfoxide, a major metabolite of chlorpromazine. A comparison with chlorpromazine*. J. Pharmacol. exp. Ther. **118**, 328—337 (1956).

—, and B. Westerholm: *The influence of reserpine on 5-hydroxytryptamine and histamine content of rat mast cells and of some rat tissues*. Acta physiol. scand. **58**, 20—29 (1963).

Morillo, A., A. M. Revzin, and T. Knauss: *Physiological mechanisms of action of chlordiazepoxide in cats*. Psychopharmacologia **3**, 386—394 (1962).

Morpurgo, C.: *Drug-induced modifications of discriminated avoidance behavior in rats*. Psychopharmacologia **8**, 91—99 (1965).

Moyer, J. H.: *The pharmacology of chlorpromazine*. J. clin. exp. Psychopath. **16**, 179—190 (1955).

Müller, J. M., E. Schlittler u. H. J. Bein: *Reserpin, der sedative Wirkstoff aus Rauwolfia serpentina Benth*. Experientia **8**, 338 (1952).

Muscholl, E., and M. Vogt: *The action of reserpine on sympathetic ganglia*. J. Physiol. **136**, 7 P (1957 a).

— — *The concentration of adrenaline in the plasma of reserpinized rabbits*. Brit. J. Pharmacol. **12**, 532—535 (1957 b).

— — *The action of reserpine on the peripheral sympathetic system*. J. Physiol. **141**, 132—155 (1958).

— *Die Wirkung von Harmalin auf die Konzentration von Noradrenalin und Adrenalin im Herzen*. Experientia **15**, 428—429 (1959).

— *Die Hemmung der Noradrenalin-Aufnahme des Herzens durch Reserpin und die Wirkung von Tyramin*. Naunyn-Schmiedeberg Arch. exp. Path. **240**, 234 bis 241 (1960).

— *Akute Hypertonie nach Monoaminoxydase-Hemmstoffen und Genuß von Käse*. Dtsch. med. Wschr. **90**, 38—39 (1965).

Naess, K., and S. Schanche: *Effect of reserpine on 5-hydroxytryptamine (serotonin) in rabbit serum*. Acta Pharmacol. **12**, 406—410 (1956).

Nakajima, T., Y. Kakimoto, and I. Sano: *Formation of β-Phenylethylamine in mammalian tissue and its effect on motor activity in the mouse*. J. Pharmacol. exp. Ther. **143**, 319—325 (1964).

Nash, C. W., E. Costa, and B. B. Brodie: *Stereospecificity in the release of H^3-NE from rat hearts by D- and L-isomers of NE*. Pharmacologist **5**, 258 (1963).

Nasmyth, P. A.: *The effect of chlorpromazine on adrenocortical activity in stress*. Brit. J. Pharmacol. **10**, 336—339 (1955).

Neff, N. H., and E. Costa: *Effect of tricyclic antidepressants and chlorpromazine on brain catecholamine synthesis*. In: Antidepressant drugs. Eds. S. Garattini and M. N. G. Dukes. Amsterdam: Excerpta Medica Fdn. 1967, pp. 28—34.

Ngai, S. H., D. T. C. Tseng, and S. C. Wang: *Effect of diazepam and other central nervous system depressants on spinal reflexes in cats: a study of site of action*. J. Pharmacol. exp. Ther. **153**, 344—351 (1966).

Niemegeers, C. J. E., and P. A. J. Janssen: *A comparative study of the inhibitory effects of haloperidol and trifluperidol on learned shock-avoidance behavioral habits and on apomorphine-induced emesis in mongrel dogs and in beagles*. Psychopharmacologia **8**, 263—270 (1965).

Norton, S, and E. J. De Beer: *Effects of drugs on the behavioral patterns of cats.* Ann. N. Y. Acad. Sci. 65, 249—257 (1956).

Oates, J. A., P. A. Nierenberg, B. Jepson, A. Sjoerdsma, and S. Undenfriend: *Conversion of phenylalanine to phenylethylamine in patients with phenylketonuria.* Proc. Soc. exp. Biol. Med. 112, 1078—1081 (1963).

Olds, J., K. F. Killam, and P. Bach-Y-Rita: *Self-stimulation of the brain used as a screening method for tranquilizing drugs.* Science 124, 265—266 (1956).

— —, and S. Eiduson: *Effects of tranquilizers on self-stimulation of the brain.* In: Psychotropic drugs. Eds. S. Garattini and V. Ghetti. Amsterdam: Elsevier Publ. Co. 1957, pp. 235—243.

— *Self-stimulation of the brain. Its use to study local effects of hunger, sex and drugs.* Science 127, 315—324 (1958).

—, and M. E. Olds: *Positive reinforcement produced by stimulating hypothalamus with iproniazid and other compounds.* Science 127, 1175—1176 (1958).

Orlans, F. B., K. F. Finger, and B. B. Brodie: *Pharmacological consequences of the selective release of peripheral norepinephrine by syrosingopine (SU 3118).* J. Pharmacol. exp. Ther. 128, 131—139 (1960).

Owen, J. E., and R. C. Rathbun: *Sustained changes of avoidance behavior after chronic nortriptyline administration.* Psychopharmacologia 9, 137—145 (1966).

Paasonen, M. K., and M. Vogt: *The effects of drugs on the amounts of substance P and 5-hydroxytryptamine in mammalian brain.* J. Physiol. 131, 617—626 (1956).

—, and O. Krayer: *The release of norepinephrine from the mammalian heart by reserpine.* J. Pharmacol. exp. Ther. 123, 153—160 (1958).

Paoletti, R., and R. Vertua: *Drugs affecting the sympathetic regulation of lipid transport.* In: Comparative Neurochemistry. Ed. D. Richter. Oxford-London-New York-Paris: Pergamon Press 1964, pp. 413—424.

Paton, W. D. M.: *Diskussionsbemerkung.* In: Adrenergic Mechanisms. Eds. J. R. Vane, G. E. W. Wolstenholme, and M. O'Connor. London: Churchill Ltd. 1960, pp. 124—127.

Penaloza-Rojas, J. H., G. Bach-Y-Rita, H. F. Rubio-Chevannier, and R. Hernández-Peón: *Effects of imipramine upon hypothalamic and amygdaloid excitability.* Exp. Neurol. 4, 205—213 (1961).

Pepeu, G., M. Roberts, S. Schanberg, and N. J. Giarman: *Differential action of iproniazid (Marsilid) and beta-phenyl-iso-propylhydrazine (Catron) on isolated atria.* J. Pharmacol. 132, 131—138 (1961).

Philippu, A., u. H. J. Schümann: *Die Bedeutung der Ribonucleinsäure für die Brenzcatechinamin- und ATP-Speicherung in den chromaffinen Granula des Nebennierenmarks.* Naunyn-Schmiedeberg Arch. exp. Path. 246, 7—8 (1963).

Piala, J. J., J. P. High, G. J. Hassert, Jr., J. C. Burke, and B. N. Craver: *Pharmacological and acute toxicological comparisons of triflupromazine and chlorpromazine.* J. Pharmacol. exp. Ther. 127, 55—65 (1959).

Pisano, J. J., J. A. Oates, Jr., A. Karmen, A. Sjoerdsma, and S. Udenfriend: *Identification of p-hydroxy-α-(methylaminomethyl)benzyl alcohol (synephrine) in human urine.* J. Biol. Chem. 236, 898—901 (1961).

Pisciotta, A. V., and J. Kaldahl: *Studies on agranulocytosis, IV. Effects of chlorpromazine on nucleic acid synthesis of bone marrow cells in vitro.* Blood 20, 781—782 (1962).

Pletscher, A., P. A. Shore, and B. B. Brodie: *Serotonin release as a possible mechanism of reserpine action.* Science 122, 374—375 (1955).

— *Beeinflussung des 5-Hydroxytryptaminstoffwechsels im Gehirn durch Isonikotinsäure-hydrazide.* Experientia 12, 479—480 (1956 a).

145

— Wirkung von Isonikotinsäurehydraziden auf den 5-Hydroxytryptaminstoffwechsel in vivo. Helv. physiol. Pharmacol. Acta 14, C 76—C 79 (1956 b).

—, P. A. Shore, and B. B. Brodie: Serotonin as a mediator of reserpine action in brain. J. Pharmacol. exp. Ther. 116, 84—89 (1956).

— Wirkung von Isopropyl-isonicotinsäurehydrazid auf den Stoffwechsel von Katecholaminen und 5-Hydroxytryptamin im Gehirn. Schweiz. med. Wschr. 87, 1532 (1957 a).

— Alteration of some biochemical and pharmacological effects of reserpine by iproniazid. In: Psychotropic drugs. Eds. S. Garattini and V. Ghetti. Amsterdam: Elsevier Publ. Co. 1957 b, pp. 468—469.

— Einfluß von Isopropyl-isonicotinsäurehydrazid auf den Katecholamingehalt des Myocards. Experientia 14, 73—74 (1958).

—, and A. Bernstein: Increase of 5-hydroxytryptamine in blood platelets by isopropyl-isonicotinic acid hydrazide. Nature 181, 1133 (1958).

—, H. Besendorf u. H. P. Bächtold: Benzo(a)chinolizine, eine neue Körperklasse mit Wirkung auf den 5-Hydroxytryptamin- und Noradrenalin-Stoffwechsel des Gehirns. Naunyn-Schmiedeberg Arch. exp. Path. 232, 499—506 (1958).

— Antagonism between harmaline and long-acting monoamine oxidase inhibitors concerning the effect on 5-hydroxytryptamine and norepinephrine metabolism in the brain. Experientia 15, 25—29 (1959).

—, and K. T. Gey: Pharmacologische Beeinflussung des 5-Hydroxytryptamin-Stoffwechsels im Gehirn und Monoaminoxydasehemmung in vitro. Helv. physiol. Acta 17, C 35—C 39 (1959).

—, H. H. Besendorf, H. P. Bächtold u. K. F. Gey: Über pharmakologische Beeinflussung des Zentralnervensystems durch kurzwirkende Monoaminoxydasehemmer aus der Gruppe der Harmala-Alkaloide. Helv. physiol. pharmacol. Acta 17, 202—214 (1959 a).

— —, and K. F. Gey: Depression of norepinephrine and 5-hydroxytryptamine in the brain by benzoquinolizine derivatives. Science 129, 844 (1959 b).

—, and K. F. Gey: Wirkung von Chlorpromazin auf pharmakologische Veränderungen des 5-Hydroxytryptamin- und Noradrenalin-Gehaltes im Gehirn. Med. exp. 2, 259—265 (1960).

— —, and P. Zeller: Monoaminoxydasehemmer. In: Fortschritte der Arzneimittelforschung, Vol. II. Basel-Stuttgart: Birkhäuser 1960, pp. 417—590.

— — Action of imipramine and amitriptyline on cerebral monoamines are compared with chlorpromazine. Med. exp. 6, 165—168 (1962).

—, E. Kunz, H. Staebler, and K. F. Gey: The uptake of tryptamine by brain in vivo and its alteration by drugs. Biochem. Pharmacol. 12, 1065—1070 (1963).

—, and M. Da Prada: Mechanism of action of neuroleptics. In: Neuropsychopharmacology, Proceedings of the Fifth International Congress, Washington, D. C. Eds. H. Brill et al. Amsterdam: Excerpta Med. Fdn. 1967, pp. 304—311.

— —, and G. Foglar: Differences between neuroleptics and tranquilizers regarding metabolism and biochemical effects. In: Neuropsychopharmacology, Proc. of the Fifth Int.'1. Cong., Washington, D. C., Eds. H. Brill et al. Amsterdam: Excerpta Medica Fdn. 1967, pp. 101—107.

Plotnikoff, N., and G. M. Everett: Potentiation of evoked cortical responses in the rabbit by methamphetamine and antidepressants. Life Sci. 4, 1135—1147 (1965).

Plummer, A. J., A. Earl, J. A. Schneider, J. Trapold, and W. Barrett: Pharmacology of rauwolfia alkaloids, including reserpine. Ann. N.Y. Acad. Sci. 59, 8—21 (1954).

—, H. Sheppard, and A. R. Schulert: The metabolism of reserpine. In: Psychotropic drugs. Eds. S. Garattini and V. Ghetti. Amsterdam: Elsevier Publ. Co. 1957, pp. 350—362.

Pöldinger, W.: *Combined administration of desipramine and reserpine or tetrabenazine in depressive patients.* Psychopharmacologia **4**, 308—310 (1963).

—, u. P. Schmidlin: *Index psychopharmacorum.* Bern-Stuttgart: H. Huber 1963.

Poirier, L. J., and T. L. Sourkes: *Influence of the substantia nigra on the catecholamine content of the striatum.* Brain **88**, 181—192 (1965).

Posner, H. S.: *Metabolism of the phenothiazine tranquilizers in humans.* In: Abstracts of papers, 136th Meeting, American Chemical Society, Atlantic City, N. J., 13—18, 1959, p. 81 C.

Preston, J. B.: *Effects of chlorpromazine on the central nervous system of the cat: a possible neural basis for action.* J. Pharmacol. exp. Ther. **118**, 100—115 (1956).

Prockop, D. J., P. A. Shore, and B. B. Brodie: *Anticonvulsant properties of monoamine oxidase inhibitors.* Ann. N. Y. Acad. Sci. **80**, 643—650 (1959).

Prusoff, W. H.: *The distribution of 5-hydroxytryptamine and adenosinetriphosphate in cytoplasmic particles of the dog's small intestine.* Brit. J. Pharmacol. **15**, 520—524 (1960).

Pscheidt, G. R., W. G. Steiner, and H. E. Himwich: *An electroencephalographic and chemical re-evaluation of the central action of reserpine in the rabbit.* J. Pharmacol. exp. Ther. **144**, 37—44 (1964).

Quastel, H. J.: *Enzymatic mechanisms of the brain and the effects of some neurotropic agents.* In: Biochemistry of the central nervous system. Ed. F. Brücke. London-New York-Paris-Los Angeles: Pergamon Press 1959, pp. 90—114.

Quinn, G. P., P. A. Shore, and B. B. Brodie: *Biochemical and pharmacological studies of RO 1—9569 (Tetrabenazine), a non-indole tranquilizing agent with reserpine-like effects.* J. Pharmacol. exp. Ther. **127**, 103—109 (1959).

Raitt, J. R., J. W. Nelson, and A. Tye: *Effect of chlorpromazine on septal hyperactivity in the rat.* Brit. J. Pharmacol. **17**, 473—478 (1961).

Randall, L. O.: *Pharmacology of methaminodiazepoxide.* Dis. nerv. Syst. **21**, 7—10 (1960).

—, W. Schallek, G. A. Heise, E. F. Keith, and R. Bagdon. *The psychosedative properties of methaminodiazepoxide.* J. Pharmacol. exp. Ther. **129** (2), 163 to 171 (1960).

—, G. A. Heise, W. Schallek, R. E. Bagdon, R. Banziger, A. Boris, R. A. Moe, and W. B. Abrams. *Pharmacological and clinical studies on Valium®—a new psychotherapeutic agent of the benzodiazepine class.* Curr. Ther. Res. **3** (9), 405—425 (1961).

—, C. L. Scheckel, and R. F. Banziger: *Pharmacology of the metabolites of chlordiazepoxide and diazepam.* Curr. Ther. Res. **7**, 590—606 (1965).

Rathbun, R. C., and I. H. Slater: *Amitriptyline and nortriptyline as antagonists of central and peripheral cholinergic activation.* Psychopharmacologia **4**, 114 to 125 (1963).

Réquin, S., J. Lanoir, R. Plas et R. Naquet: *Etude comparative des effects neurophysiologiques du Librium et du Valium.* C. R. Soc. Biol. (Paris) **157**, 2015 to 2019 (1963).

Richter, D.: *Biochemical mechanisms related to the site of action of psychotropic drugs.* In: Neuropsychopharmacology, Vol. II. Ed. E. Rothlin. Amsterdam: Elsevier Publ. Co. 1961, pp. 422—434.

Riley, H, and A. Spinks: *Biological assessment of tranquilizers.* J. Pharm. Pharmacol. **10**, 657—671 (1958).

Rinaldi, F., and H. E. Himwich: *Drugs affecting psychotic behavior and the function of the mesodiencephalic activating system.* Dis. nerv. Syst. **16**, 133—142 (1955 a).

Rinaldi F., and H. E. Himwich: *A comparison of effects of reserpine and some barbiturates on the electrical activity of cortical and subcortical structures of the brain of rabbits.* Ann. N. Y. Acad. Sci. 61, 27—35 (1955 b).

Roldan, E., and A. Escobar: *Control of convulsive activity and the effects on afferent transmission produced by methaminodiazepoxide: experimental study in the cat.* Bol. Inst. Estud. Med. Biol. (Mex.) 19, 125—153 (1961).

Roos, B.-E., and B. Werdinius: *Effect of reserpine on the level of 5-hydroxyindole-acetic acid in brain.* Life Sci. 1, 105—107 (1962).

—, and G. Steg: *The effect of L-3,4-dihydroxyphenylalanine and DL-5-hydroxy-tryptophan on rigidity and tremor induced by reserpine, chlorpromazine and phenoxybenzamine.* Life Sci. 3, 351—360 (1964).

— *Effects of certain tranquillizers on the level of homovanillic acid in the corpus striatum.* J. Pharm. Pharmacol. 17, 820—821 (1965).

Rosengren, E.: *On the role of monoamine oxidase for the inactivation of dopamine in brain.* Acta physiol. scand. 49, 370—375 (1960).

Rosenkilde, H., and W. M. Govier: *A comparison of some phenothiazine derivatives in inhibiting apomorphine-induced emesis.* J. Pharmacol. exp. Ther. 120, 375—378 (1957).

Rossiter, R. J.: *Lipid metabolism.* In: Metabolism of the nervous system. Ed. D. Richter. London-New York-Paris-Los Angeles: Pergamon Press 1957, pp. 355 to 379.

Roth, F. E., S. Irwin, E. Eckhardt, I. I. A. Tabachnik, and W. M. Govier: *Perphenazine (Trilafon), an new potent tranquilizer and antiemetic: II. General pharmacology.* Arch. int. Pharmacodyn. 118, 375—383 (1959).

Roth, G.: *Psychopharmakon, hoc est: medicina animae (1548).* Confin. Psychiat. (Basel) 7, 179—182 (1964).

Rothballer, A. B.: *The effects of catecholamines on the central nervous system.* Pharmacol. Rev. 11, 494—547 (1959).

Rubio-Chevannier, H., G. Bach-Y-Rita, J. Penaloza-Rojas, and R. Hernández-Peón: *Potentiating action of imipramine upon reticular arousal.* Exp. Neurol. 4, 214—220 (1961).

Rummel, W.: *Vergleichende Untersuchung Serotonin-, Adrenalin- und Histamin-antagonistischer Eigenschaften von Phenothiazinderivaten am terminalen Ileum des Meerschweinchens.* Med. exp. 4, 126—134 (1961).

Ryall, R. W.: *Some actions of chlorpromazine.* Brit. J. Pharmacol. 11, 339—345 (1956).

Sabelli, H., J. Levin, and J. Toman: *Interactions of imipramine and autonomic agents.* Fed. Proc. 20, 393 (1961).

Sacra, P., and J. D. MacColl: *Effect of ataractics on some convulsant and de-pressant agents in mice.* Arch. int. Pharmacodyn. 117, 1—8 (1958).

Sadove, M. S., M. J. Levin, R. Rose, and L. Schwartz: *Chlorpromazine and nar-cotics in the management of pain of malignant disease.* J. Amer. med. Ass. 155, 626—628 (1954).

—, R. C. Balagot, and J. M. McGrath: *Effects of chlordiazepoxide and diazepam on the influence of meperidine on the respiratory response to carbon dioxide.* J. New drugs 5, 121—124 (1965).

Safran, M., and M. Vogt: *Depletion of pituitary corticotrophin by reserpine and by a nitrogen mustard.* Brit. J. Pharmacol. 15, 165—169 (1960).

Sailer, S., u. Ch. Stumpf: *Reserpinwirkung auf das Kaninchen-EEG.* Arch. exp. Path. Pharmakol. 230, 378—385 (1957).

Salzman, N. P., and B. B. Brodie: *Physiological disposition and fate of chlor-promazine and a method for its estimation in biological material.* J. Pharmacol. exp. Ther. 118, 46—54 (1956).

Sanan, S., and M. Vogt: *Effect of drugs on the noradrenaline content of brain and peripheral tissues and its significance.* Brit. J. Pharmacol. 18, 109—127 (1962).

Sandberg, F.: *A comparative quantitative study of the central depressant effect of seven clinically used phenothiazine derivatives.* Arzneimittel-Forsch. 9, 203 to 206 (1959).

Sano, I., T. Gamo, Y. Kakimoto, K. Taniguchi, M. Takesada, and K. Nishinuma: *Distribution of catechol compounds in human brain.* Biochem. biophys. Acta 32, 586—587 (1959).

Satanove, A.: *Pigmentation due to phenothiazines in high and prolonged dosage.* J. Amer. med. Ass. 191, 263—268 (1965).

Schallek, W., A. Kuehn, and D. K. Seppelin: *Central depressant effects of methyprylon.* J. Pharmacol. exp. Ther. 118, 139—147 (1956).

— —, and N. Jew: *Effects of chlordiazepoxide (Librium) and other psychotropic agents on the limbic system of the brain.* Ann. N. Y. Acad. Sci. 96, 303—314 (1962).

—, F. Zabransky, and A. Kuehn: *Effects of benzodiazepines on central nervous system of cat.* Arch. int. Pharmacodyn. 149, 467—483 (1964).

Schanberg, S., and N. J. Giarman: *Drug-induced alterations in the subcellular distribution of 5-hydroxytryptamine.* Biochem. Pharmacol. 11, 187—194 (1962).

—, J. J. Schildkraut, and I. J. Kopin: *The effects of psychoactive drugs on norepinephrine-H³ metabolism in brain.* Biochem. Pharmacol. 16, 393—399 (1967).

Schaumann, W.: *Beeinflussung der analgetischen Wirkung des Morphins durch Reserpin.* Naunyn-Schmiedeberg Arch. exp. Path. 235, 1—9 (1958).

Scheckel, C. L., and E. Boff: *Behavioral effects of interacting imipramine and other drugs with d-amphetamine, cocaine and tetrabenazine.* Psychopharmacologia 5, 198—208 (1964).

Scheel-Krüger, J., and A. Randrup: *Stereotyped hyperactive behavior produced by dopamine in the absence of noradrenaline.* Life Sci. 6, 1389—1398 (1967).

Schenker, E., u. H. Herbst: *Phenothiazine und Azaphenothiazine als Heilmittel.* In: Fortschritte der Arzneimittelforschung, Vol. V. Ed. E. Jucker. Basel-Stuttgart: Birkhäuser Verlag 1963, pp. 269—627.

Schimmerl, G., and Ch. Stumpf: *Die Tätigkeit des nucleus ruber nach Verabreichung von Barbituraten und Meprobamat.* Arch. exp. Path. Pharmakol. 235, 30—40 (1958).

Schmid, E., L. Zicha, F. Scheiffarth u. O. Büttner: *Untersuchungen über den Antagonismus von Antihistaminen und Serotonin.* Arzneimittel-Forsch. 9, 474—476 (1959).

Schmidt, R. F., M. E. Vogel, and M. Zimmerman: *The effect of diazepam on presynaptic inhibition and other spinal cord reflexes.* Arch. exp. Path. Pharmakol. 258, 69—82 (1967).

Schmitt, H., and H. Schmitt: *Valeur de la pharmacologie prévisionelle dans le domaine des antidépresseurs dérivés de l'iminodibenzyle.* Thérapie 21, 653—674 (1966 a).

— — *Inhibition de l'hypertension réserpinique postamphetaminique par les substances antidépressives du groupe de l'imipramine.* C. R. Soc. Biol. 160, 303—306 (1966 b).

— *Selective actions of antidepressant drugs on some rhinencephalic and related structures.* In: Antidepressant drugs. Eds. G. Garattini and M. N. G. Dukes. Amsterdam: Excerpta Medica Fdn. 1967, pp. 104—115.

—, et P. Gonnard: *Modifications par un inhibiteur de l'aminoxydase, l'iproniazide, des effects de quelques amines sympathicomimétiques sur la membrane nictitante du chat.* Arch. int. Pharmacodyn. 108, 74—83 (1956).

149

Schmitt, H., et H. Schmitt: *Action de la chlorpromazine sur les centres vasomoteurs.* Arch. int. Pharmacodyn. **132**, 74—90 (1961).

— — *Cardiovascular actions of haloperidol.* Arch. int. Pharmacodyn. **137**, 91—107 (1962).

Schneider, J. A.: *Reserpine antagonism of morphine analgesia in mice.* Proc. Soc. exp. Biol. Med. **87**, 614—615 (1954).

—, and A. E. Earl: *Behavioral and electroencephalographic studies with Serpasil (reserpine), a new alkaloid from rauwolfia serpentina B.* Fed. Proc. **13**, 130 (1954).

—, A. J. Plummer, A. E. Earl, and R. Gaunt: *Neuropharmacological aspects of reserpine.* Ann. N. Y. Acad. **61**, 17—26 (1955).

—, and R. K. Rinehart: *Circulatory interactions of serotonin and reserpine (serpasil) in dogs.* Arch. int. Pharmacodyn. **105**, 253—268 (1956).

Schneidman, E. S., N. L. Farberow, and C. V. Leonard: cit. L. Hollister (1964).

Schümann, H. J.: *Über den Noradrenalin- und ATP-Gehalt sympathischer Nerven.* Naunyn-Schmiedeberg Arch. exp. Path. **233**, 296—300 (1958 a).

— *Die Wirkung von Insulin und Reserpin auf den Adrenalin- und ATP-Gehalt der chromaffinen Granula des Nebennierenmarks.* Naunyn-Schmiedeberg Arch. exp. Path. **233**, 237—249 (1958 b).

— *Über den Hydroxytyramingehalt der Organe.* Naunyn-Schmiedeberg Arch. exp. Path. **236**, 474—482 (1959).

—, u. A. Philippu: *Untersuchungen zum Mechanismus der Freisetzung von Brenz-catechinaminen durch Tyramin.* Naunyn-Schmiedeberg Arch. exp. Path. **241**, 273—280 (1961).

Schwartz, M. A., B. A. Koechlin, E. Postma, S. Palmer, and G. Krol: *Metabolism of diazepam in rat, dog, and man.* J. Pharmacol. exp. Ther. **149**, 423—435 (1965).

Scott, G. T., and L. K. Nading: *Relative effectiveness of phenothiazine tranquilizing drugs causing release of MSH.* Proc. Soc. exp. Biol. Med. **106**, 88—90 (1961).

Scriabine, A., and M. Blake: *Evaluation of centrally acting drugs in mice with fighting behavior induced by isolation.* Psychopharmacologia **3**, 224—226 (1962).

Seeman, P. M., and H. S. Bialy: *The surface activity of tranquilizers.* Biochem. Pharmacol. **12**, 1181—1191 (1963).

Seiden, L. S., and A. Carlsson: *Temporary and partial antagonism by L-DOPA of reserpine-induced suppression of a conditioned avoidance response.* Psychopharmacologia **4**, 418—423 (1963).

— — *Brain and heart catecholamine levels after L-DOPA administration in reserpine treated mice: Correlations with a conditioned avoidance response.* Psychopharmacologia **5**, 178—181 (1964).

—, and L. C. F. Hanson: *Reversal of the reserpine-induced suppression of the conditioned avoidance response in the cat by L-DOPA.* Psychopharmacologia **6**, 239—244 (1964).

Seitelberger, F., H. Petsche, H. Bernheimer u. O. Hornykiewicz: *Verhalten des Dopamins (= 3-Hydroxytyramin) im Nucleus caudatus nach elektrischer Koagulation des Globus pallidus.* Naturwissenschaften **5**, 314—315 (1964).

Shagass, C.: *Effect of intravenous chlorpromazine on the electroencephalogram.* Electroenceph. clin. Neurophysiol. **7**, 306 (1955).

Sharman, D. F.: *Changes in the metabolism of 3,4-dihydroxyphenyl-ethylamine (dopamine) in the striatum of the mouse induced by drugs.* Brit. J. Pharmacol. **28**, 153—163 (1966).

Sheppard, H., R. A. Lucas, and W. H. Tsien: *The metabolism of reserpine-C^{14}.* Arch. int. Pharmacodyn. **103**, 256—269 (1955).

Shimizu, A., Y. Hishikawa, K. Matsumoto, and Z. Kaneko: *Electroencephalographic studies on the action of monoamine oxidase inhibitor.* Psychopharmacologia 6, 368—387 (1964).

Shore, P. A., A. Pletscher, E. G. Tomich, R. Kuntzman, and B. B. Brodie: *Release of blood platelet serotonin by reserpine and lack of effect on bleeding time.* J. Pharmacol. exp. Ther. 117, 232—236 (1956 a).

—, A. Carlsson, and B. B. Brodie: *Mechanism of serotonin-release by reserpine.* Fed. Proc. 15, 483 (1956 b).

—, L. Gillespie, S. Spector, and D. Prockop: *Increase of blood serotonin levels induced by iproniazid in man and rabbits.* Naturwissenschaften 45, 340—341 (1958).

Sigg, E. B., and J. A. Schneider: *Mechanisms involved in the interaction of various central stimulants and reserpine.* EEG and Clin. Neurophysiol. J. 9, 419—426 (1957).

—, G. Carpio, and J. A. Schneider: *Synergism of amines and antagonism of reserpine to morphine analgesia.* Proc. Soc. exp. Biol. Med. 97, 97—100 (1958).

— *Pharmacological studies with Tofranil.* Canad. Psychiat. Ass. J. 4 (Suppl.), 75—85 (1959).

—, L. Soffer, and L. Gyermek: *Influence of imipramine and related psychoactive agents on the effect of 5-hydroxytryptamine and catecholamines on the cat nictitating membrane.* J. Pharmacol. exp. Ther. 142, 13—20 (1963).

—, L. Gyermek, and R. Hill: *Antagonism to reserpine-induced depression by imipramine, related psychoactive drugs and some autonomic agents.* Psychopharmacologia 7, 144—149 (1965).

—, and R. Hill: *The effect of imipramine on central adrenergic mechanisms.* In: Neuropsychopharmacology, Proc. V. Int'l. Congress CINP, Washington, D. C. (1966). Amsterdam: Excerpta Medica Fdn. 1967.

Silvestrini, B., and G. Maffii: *Effects of chlorpromazine, promazine, diethazine, reserpine, hydroxyzine, and morphine upon some mono- and polysynaptic motor reflexes.* J. Pharm. Pharmacol. 11, 224—233 (1959).

Sjoerdsma, A., W. Lovenberg, J. A. Oates, J. R. Crout, and S. Udenfriend: *Alterations in the pattern of amine excretion in man produced by a monoamine oxidase inhibitor.* Science 130, 225 (1959 a).

—, J. A. Oates, P. Zaltzman, and S. Udenfriend: *Identification and assay of urinary tryptamine; application as an index of monoamine oxidase inhibition in man.* J. Pharmacol. exp. Ther. 126, 217—222 (1959 b).

— —, and L. Gillespie: *Quantitation of monoamine oxidase inhibition produced with various drugs in man.* Proc. Soc. exp. Biol. Med. 103, 485—487 (1960).

Sjöqvist, F.: *Interaction between monoamine oxidase (MAO) inhibitors and other substances.* Proc. roy. Soc. Med. 58, 967—978 (1965).

—, and J. Gillette: *Prolongation and potentiation of oxotremorine effects of DMI, an "antitremorine" drug.* Life Sci. 4, 1031—1036 (1965).

Slater, I. H., R. C. Rathbun, F. G. Henderson, and N. Neuss: *Pharmacological properties of recanescine, a new sedative alkaloid from rauwolfia canescens Linn.* Proc. Soc. exp. Biol. Med. 88, 292—295 (1955).

Smith, C. B.: *Enhancement by reserpine and α-methyl-dopa of the effects of d-amphetamine upon the locomotor activity of mice.* J. Pharmacol. exp. Ther. 142, 343—350 (1963).

Soudijn, W., I. Van Wijngaarden, and F. Allewijn: *Distribution, excretion and metabolism of neuroleptics of the butyrophenone type.* Europ. J. Pharmacol. 1, 47—57 (1967).

Spector, S., R. Kuntzman, P. A. Shore, and B. B. Brodie: *Evidence for release of brain amines by reserpine in presence of monoamine oxidase inhibitors: implication of monoamine oxidase in norepinephrine metabolism in brain.* J. Pharmacol. exp. Ther. 130, 256—261 (1960 a).

—, P. A. Shore, and B. B. Brodie: *Biochemical and pharmacological effect of monoamine oxidase inhibitors, iproniazid, 1-phenyl-2-hydrazinopropan (JB-516) and 1-phenyl-3-hydrazinobutane (JB-835).* J. Pharmacol. exp. Ther. 128, 15—21 (1960 b).

—, A. Sjoerdsma, and S. Udenfriend: *Blockade of endogenous norepinephrine synthesis by α-methyltyrosine, an inhibitor of tyrosine hydroxylase.* J. Pharmacol. exp. Ther. 147, 86—95 (1965).

Spencer, P. S. J.: *Activity of centrally acting and other drugs against tremor and hypothermia induced in mice by tremorine.* Brit. J. Pharmacol. 25, 442—455 (1965).

Spiegel, E. A., and E. G. Szekely: *Prolonged stimulation of the head of the caudate nucleus.* Arch. Neurol. 4, 67—77 (1961).

Spirtes, M. A., and P. S. Guth: *An effect of chlorpromazine on rat mitochondrial membranes.* Nature 190, 274—275 (1961).

— — *Effects of chlorpromazine on biological membranes I. Chlorpromazine-induced changes in liver.* Biochem. Pharmacol. 12, 37—46 (1963).

Stacey, R. S.: *Uptake of 5-hydroxytryptamine by platelets.* Brit. J. Pharmacol. 16, 284—295 (1961).

Staehelin, J. E., u. P. Kielholtz: *Largactil, ein neues vegetatives Dämpfungsmittel bei psychischen Störungen.* Schweiz. med. Wschr. 83, 581—586 (1953).

Starbuck, W. C., and H. C. Heim: *Some in vitro effects of chlorpromazine, lysergic acid diethylamide and 5-hydroxytryptamine on the respiration of rat brain.* J. Amer. pharm. Ass. (Sci. Ed.) 48, 251—253 (1959).

Stark, P., and J. K. Henderson: *Differentiation of classes of neurosedatives using rats with septal lesions.* Int. J. Neuropharmacol. 5, 385—389 (1966).

Steg, G.: *α-Rigidity in reserpinized rats.* Experientia 29, 79—80 (1964).

Stein, L., and J. Seifter: *Possible mode of antidepressive action of imipramine.* Science 134, 286—287 (1961).

Sternbach, L. H., L. O. Randall, and S. R. Gustafson: *1,4-Benzodiazepines (Chlordiazepoxide and related compounds).* Ed. M. Gordon, Vol. I. New York: Academic Press 1964, p. 137.

Stjärne, L., and S. Schapiro: *Effects of reserpine on secretion from the adrenal medulla.* Nature 182, 1450 (1958).

— *Studies of catecholamine uptake, storage and release mechanisms.* Acta Physiol. scand. 62 (Suppl.), 228 (1964).

Stock, K., u. E. Westermann: *Biogene Amine im Fettgewebe.* Naunyn-Schmiedeberg Arch. exp. Path. 246, 15—16 (1963).

Stone, G. C., B. M. Bernstein, W. E. Hambourger, and V. A. Drill: *Behavioral and pharmacological studies of thiopropazate, a potent tranquilizing agent.* Arch. int. Pharmacodyn. 127, 85—103 (1960).

Stumpf, Ch.: In: Handbuch der exper. Pharmakologie. Bd. 16: *Erzeugung von Krankheitszuständen durch das Experiment.* Teil 7: *Zentralnervensystem.* Pharmakologische Methoden. Berlin-Göttingen-Heidelberg: Springer 1962, pp. 1—105.

Sulman, F. G.: *The mammotropic effect of ataractic drugs.* Biochem. Pharmacol. 8, 101—102 (1961).

Sulser, F., J. Watts, and B. B. Brodie: *Antagonistic action of imipramine and reserpine on central nervous system.* Fed. Proc. 19, 268 (1960).

Sulser, F., M. H. Bickel, and B. B. Brodie: *The action of desmethylimipramine in counteracting sedation and cholinergic effects of reserpine-like drugs.* J. Pharmacol. exp. Ther. 144, 321—330 (1964).

—, M. L. Owens, and J. V. Dingell: *On the mechanism of amphetamine potentiation by desipramine (DMI).* Life Sci. 5, 2005—2010 (1966).

Suzuki, M., K. Kamio, M. Yasuda, S. Akiyama, K. Mitani, T. Oyama, K. Sato, and T. Yamashita: *Effect of chlorpromazine on the function of the endocrine organs.* Endocr. Jap. 3, 67—72 (1956).

Swinyard, E. A., H. H. Wolf, G. B. Fink, and L. S. Goodman: *Some neuropharmacological properties of thioridazine hydrochloride (Mellaril).* J. Pharmacol. exp. Ther. 126, 312—317 (1959).

Taeschler, M., u. A. Cerletti: *Zur Pharmakologie von Thioridazin, Mellaril.* Schweiz. med. Wschr. 88, 1216—1220 (1958).

— — *Differential analysis of the effects of phenothiazine-tranquilizers on emotional and motor behavior in experimental animals.* Nature 184, 823 (1959).

—, A. Fanchamps u. A. Cerletti: *Zur Bedeutung verschiedener pharmakologischer Eigenschaften der Phenothiazinderivate für ihre klinische Wirksamkeit.* Psychiat. Neurol. (Basel) 139, 85—104 (1960).

—, and A. Cerletti: *Inhibition of emotional reactions by phenothiazine tranquilizers.* Nature 190, 1014—1015 (1961).

—, u. D. Loew: *Zur Pharmakologie der in der Kinderpsychiatrie gebräuchlichen psychotropen Medikamente.* Acta paedopsychiat. (Basel) 32 (Suppl. I), (1965).

Takaori, S., and G. A. Deneau: cit. E. F. Domino (1962 a).

Takemoto, Y., P. A. Shore, E. F. Tomich, R. Kuntzman, and B. B. Brodie: *Studies on the mechanism of reserpine-induced epinephrine release and hyperglycemia.* J. Pharmacol. exp. Ther. 119, 188 (1957).

Tangri, K. K., and K. P. Bhargava: *Localization of the central site of hypotensive action of chlorpromazine.* Arch. int. Pharmacodyn. 127, 274—284 (1960).

Tardieu, G., C. Tardieu et J. Hariga: *Action du Valium sur la rigidité décérébrée expérimentale et sur les raideurs de l'enfant infirme moteur cérébral.* Acta Neurol. Psychiat. Belg. 64, 1133—1140 (1964).

Tedeschi, D. H.: cit. C. L. Zirkle and C. Kaiser.

—, J. P. Benigni, C. J. Elder, J. C. Yeager, and J. V. Flanigau: *Effects of various phenothiazines on minimal electroshock seizure threshold and spontaneous motor activity of mice.* J. Pharmacol. exp. Ther. 123, 35—38 (1958).

—, R. E. Tedeschi, L. Cook, P. A. Mattis, and E. J. Fellows: *The neuropharmacology of trifluoperazine: A potent psychotherapeutic agent.* Arch. int. Pharmacodyn. 122, 129—143 (1959 a).

— —, and E. J. Fellows: *Effects of tryptamine on the central nervous system, including a pharmacological procedure for the evaluation of iproniazid-like drugs.* J. Pharmacol. exp. Ther. 126, 223—232 (1959 b).

— — — *Activity of various pharmacological agents as in vivo inhibitors of monoamine oxidase.* Fed. Proc. 19, 278 (1960).

Terzian, H.: *Studio elettroencefalografico dell'azione centrale del Largactil (4560 RP).* Rass. Neurol. veg. 9, 211—215 (1952).

— *Etude de l'action du largactil (4560 RP) et du pendiomide sur l'activité électrique cérébrale du lapin.* Rev. Neurol. 91, 445—453 (1954).

Theobald, W., O. Büch, H. Kunz, C. Morpurgo, E. G. Stenger, and G. Wilhelmi: *Comparative pharmacological studies with Tofranil, Pertofran and Ensidon.* Arch. int. Pharmacodyn. (Ger.) 148, 560—596 (1964).

— — — *Comparative studies of the influence of psychotropic drugs on autonomic functions in acute animal experiments.* Arzneimittelforschung (Ger.) 15, 117 to 125 (1965).

Tissot, R., et M. Monnier: *Suppression de l'action de la reserpine sur le cerveau par ses antagonistes: Iproniazid et LSD.* Helvet. physiol. Acta 16, 268—276 (1958).

Tokizane, T., M. Kawakami, and E. Gellhorn: *Pharmacological investigations on the antagonism between the activating and recruiting systems.* Arch. int. Pharmacodyn. 113, 217—232 (1957).

Toman, J. E. P.: *Some aspects of central nervous pharmacology.* Ann. Rev. Pharmacol. 3, 153—184 (1963).

Trendelenburg, U.: *Modification of the effect of tyramine by various agents and procedures.* J. Pharmacol. exp. Ther. 134, 8—17 (1961).

— *Supersensitivity and subsensitivity to sympathomimetic amines.* Pharmacol. Rev. 15, 225—276 (1963).

—, and J. S. Gravenstein: *Effect of reserpine pretreatment on stimulation of the accelerans nerve of the dog.* Science 128, 901—902 (1958).

Tripod, J., H. I. Bein, and R. Meier: *Characterization of central effects of Serpasil (Reserpine-a new alkaloid of Rauwolfia serpentina B.) and of their antagonistic reactions.* Arch int. Pharmacodyn. 96, 406—425 (1954).

Tuchmann-Duplessis, H., et L. Mercier-Parot: *Action de la reserpine sur l'appareil génital de la Ratte adulte.* C. R. Acad. Sci. 242, 1233—1235 (1956).

Tui, C., E. Riley, and A. Orr: *17-Hydrocorticosteroid levels in the peripheral blood of psychotic patients under treatment with chlorpromazine and reserpine: A preliminary study.* J. clin. exp. Psychopath. 17, 142—146 (1956).

Twarog, B. M., and I. H. Page: *Serotonin content of some mammalian tissues and urine and a method of its determination.* Amer. J. Physiol. 175, 157—161 (1953).

Udenfriend, S., H. Weissbach, and D. Bogdanski: *Biochemical findings related to the action of serotonin.* Ann. N. Y. Acad. Sci. 66, 602—608 (1957).

—, B. Witkop, B. G. Redfield, and D. F. Bogdanski: *Studies with reversible inhibitors of monoamine oxidase: Harmaline and related compounds.* Biochem. Pharmacol. 1, 160—165 (1958).

—, C. R. Creveling, M. Ozaki, J. W. Daly, and B. Witkop: *Inhibitors of norepinephrine metabolism in vivo.* Arch. Biochem. 84, 249—251 (1959).

Uhrbrand, L., and A. Faurbye: *Reversible and irreversible dyskinesia after treatment with perphenazine, chlorpromazine, reserpine and electroconvulsive therapy.* Psychopharmacologia 1, 408—418 (1960).

Umbach, W., u. D. Baumann: *Die Wirksamkeit von L-DOPA bei Parkinsonpatienten mit und ohne stereotaktischen Eingriff.* Arch. Psychiat. Nervenkr. 205, 281—292 (1964).

Unna, K. R., and W. R. Martin: *The action of chlorpromazine on the electrical activity of the brain.* In: Psychotropic dugs. Eds. G. Garattini and V. Ghetti. Amsterdam: Elsevier Publ. Co. 1957, pp. 272—282.

Usdin, E., and D. H. Efron: *Psychotropic drugs and related compounds.* Public Health Service Publication # 1589; Sup't. of Documents. Washington, D. C.: U. S. Gov't. Printing Office 1967.

Van der Schoot, J. B., E. J. Ariëns, J. M. Van Rossum, and J. A. T. M. Hurkmans: *Phenylisopropylamine derivatives, structure and action.* Arzneimittel-Forsch. 12, 902—907 (1962).

Vane, J. R.: *The relative activities of some tryptamine analogues on the isolated rat stomach strip preparation.* Brit. J. Pharmacol. 14, 87—98 (1959).

—, H. O. J. Collier, S. J. Corne, E. Marley, and P. B. Bradley: *Tryptamine receptors in the central nervous system.* Nature 191, 1068—1069 (1961).

Van Rossum, J. M.: *Different types of sympathomimetic α-receptors.* J. Pharm. Pharmacol. 17, 202—216 (1965).

Van Rossum, J. M.: *The significance of dopamine-receptor blockade for the mechanism of action of neuroleptic drugs.* Arch. int. Pharmacodyn. 160 (2), 492—494 (1966).

— *The significance of dopamine-receptor blockades for the action of neuroleptic drugs.* In: Neuropsychopharmacology. Proc. of the Fifth Int'l. Congress, Washington, D. C., Eds. H. Brill et al. Amsterdam: Excerpta Medica Fdn. 1967, pp. 321—329.

Van Tamelen, E. E., and P. D. Hance: *The stereochemical formulation of reserpine.* J. Amer. chem. Soc. 77, 4692—4693 (1955).

Van Zwieten, P. A., H. Bernheimer u. O. Hornykiewicz: *Zentrale Wirkung des Reserpins auf die Kreislaufreflexe des Carotissinus.* Naunyn-Schmiedeberg Arch. exp. Path. 253, 310—326 (1966).

Vernier, V., H. Hanson, and C. Stone: *The pharmacodynamics of amitriptyline.* In: Psychosomatic medicine, Chapt. 80. Eds. J. H. Nodine and J. H. Moyer. Philadelphia: Lea & Febiger 1962, pp. 683—690.

Vernier, V. G., and K. R. Unna: *Effect of stimulant drugs on tremor in monkeys.* J. Pharmacol. exp. Ther. 110, 50 (1954).

Vogt, M.: *The concentration of sympathin in different parts of the central nervous system under normal conditions and after the administration of drugs.* J. Physiol. (Lond.) 123, 451—481 (1954).

— *Distribution of adrenaline and noradrenaline in the central nervous system and its modification by drugs.* In: Metabolism of the nervous system. Ed. D. Richter. New York: Pergamon Press 1957, pp. 553—564.

— *Catecholamines in brain.* Pharmacol. Rev. 11, 483—489 (1959).

Votava, Z., J. Metysova, O. Benesova, and Z. Bohdanecky: *Comparison of pharmacological effects of some antidepressants of imipramine-type and their desmethyl derivatives.* In: Neuropsychopharmacology, Vol. IV. Eds. D. Bente and P. B. Bradley. Amsterdam: Elsevier Publ. Co. 1965, pp. 395—401.

Waalkes, T. P., and H. Weissbach: *In vivo release of histamine from rabbit blood by reserpine.* Proc. Soc. exp. Biol. Med. 93, 394—396 (1956).

— —, J. Bozicevich, and S. Udenfriend: *Further studies on release of serotonin and histamine during anaphylaxis in the rabbit.* Proc. Soc. exp. Biol. Med. 95, 479—482 (1957).

—, H. Coburn, and L. L. Terry: *The effect of reserpine on histamine and serotonine.* J. Allergy 30, 408—414 (1959).

Wagensommer, J.: *Therapeutisch unerwünschte Wirkungen der Thymoleptika.* Fortschr. Neurol. Psychiat. 32, 497—512 (1964).

Walkenstein, S. S., and J. Seifert: *Fate, distribution and excretion of S^{35} promazine.* J. Pharmacol. exp. Ther. 125, 283—286 (1959).

—, C. M. Knebel, J. A. MacMullen, and J. Seifter: *The excretion and distribution of meprobamate and its metabolites.* J. Pharmacol. exp. Ther. 123, 254—258 (1958).

Wang, H.-H., T. Kanai, S. Markee, and S. C. Wang: *Effects of reserpine and chlorpromazine on the vasomotor center in the medulla oblongata of the dog.* J. Pharmacol. exp. Ther. 144, 186—195 (1964).

Wang, S. C.: *Perphenazine, a potent and effective antiemetic.* J. Pharmacol. exp. Ther. 123, 306—310 (1958).

Ward, A. A., Jr., W. S. McCulloch, and H. W. Magoun: *Production of an alternating tremor at rest in monkeys.* J. Neurophysiol. 11, 317—330 (1948).

Watt, D. S., and T. G. Crookes: *The effect of reserpine on perceptual performance in human subjects.* In: Neuropsychopharmacology, Vol. II. Ed. E. Rothlin. Amsterdam: Elsevier Publ. Co. 1961, pp. 410—413.

Weil-Malherbe, H., and A. D. Bone: *The effect of reserpine on the intracellular distribution of catecholamines in the brain stem of the rabbit*. J. Neurochem. 4, 251—263 (1959).

—, H. S. Posner, and G. R. Bowles: *Changes in the concentration and intracellular distribution of brain catecholamines: The effects of reserpine, β-phenyliso-propylhydrazine, pyrogallol, and 3,4-dihydroxyphenylalanine, alone and in combination*. J. Pharmacol. exp. Ther. 132, 278—286 (1961).

Weiskrantz, L., and W. A. Wilson: *The effect of reserpine on emotional behavior on normal and brain operated monkeys*. Ann. N. Y. Acad. Sci. 61, 36—55 (1955).

Weissman, A., and K. F. Finger: *Effects of benzquinamide on avoidance behavior and brain amine levels*. Biochem. Pharmacol. 11, 871—880 (1962).

Werner, G.: *Clinical pharmacology of central stimulant and antidepressant drugs*. Clin. Pharmacol. Ther. 3, 59—96 (1962).

— *Zur Wirkung von Rauwolfia serpentina*. Arzneimittel-Forsch. 4, 40—41 (1954).

Westermann, E. O., R. P. Maickel, and B. B. Brodie: *Some biochemical effects of reserpine mediated by the pituitary*. Fed. Proc. 19, 268 (1960).

— *Stimulierung und Blockierung des Hypophysen-Nebennierenrinden-Systems durch Reserpin*. Naunyn-Schmiedeberg Arch. Exp. Path. 241, 518—519 (1961).

— *Cumulative effects of reserpine on the pituitary-adrenocortical and sympathetic nervous system*. In: Drugs and enzymes. Proc. II. Int'l. Pharmacol. Meeting, Prague (1963). Oxford-London-Edinburgh-New York-Paris-Frankfurt: Pergamon Press 1965, pp. 381—392.

Whitelaw, M. J.: *Delay in ovulation and menstruation induced by chlorpromazine*. J. clin. Endocr. 16, 972 (1956).

Whittaker, V. P.: cit. D. Richter.

Whitten, L. K., and D. B. Filmer: *A photosensitized keratitis in young cattle following the use of phenothiazine as an anthelmintic, I. A. clinical description with a note on its widespread occurrence in New Zealand*. Aust. Vet. J. 23, 336—340 (1947).

Wilkens, R. W.: *Clinical usage of Rauwolfia alkaloids, including reserpine (Serpasil)*. Ann. N. Y. Acad. Sci. 59, 36—44 (1954).

Williams, R. T., and D. V. Parke: *The metabolic fate of drugs*. Amer. Rev. Pharmac. 4, 85—114 (1964).

Wilson, V. J., and W. H. Talbot: *The current conditioning in the cat spinal cord: differential effect of meprobamate on recurrent facilitation and inhibition*. J. Gen. Physiology 43, 495—502 (1960).

Windsor, T.: *Control of conditioned responses of digital blood vessels*. Clin. Res. Proc. 5, 66 (1957).

Wirth, W.: *Versuche zur kombinierten Wirkung von Megaphen mit stark wirksamen Analgeticis*. Naunyn-Schmiedeberg Arch. exp. Path. 222, 75—76 (1954).

—, R. Gösswald, V. Hörlein, Kl.-H. Risse u. H. Kreiskott: *Zur Pharmakologie acylierter Phenothiazin-Derivate*. I. Mitteilung. Arch. int. Pharmacodyn. 115, 1—31 (1958).

— — u. W. Vater: *Zur Pharmakologie acylierter Phenothiazin-Derivate*. II. Mitteilung. Arch. int. Pharmacodyn. 123, 78—144 (1959).

Withrington, P., and E. Zaimis: *The reserpine-treated cat*. Brit. J. Pharmacol. 17, 380—391 (1961).

Woodson, R. E., Jr., W. W. Youngken, E. Schlittler, and J. A. Schneider: *Rauwolfia, Botany, Pharmacognosy, Chemistry and Pharmacology*. Boston-Toronto: Little, Brown 1957.

Woodward, R. B., F. E. Bader, H. Bickel, A. J. Frey, and R. W. Kirstead: *The total synthesis of reserpine*. Tetrahedron 2, 1—57 (1958).

Wooley, D. W., and E. Shaw: *A biochemical and pharmacological suggestion about certain mental disorders.* Science 119, 587—588 (1954).

— — *Evidence for the participation of serotonin in mental processes.* Ann. N. Y. Acad. Sci. 66, 649—667 (1957).

—, and P. M. Edelman: *Displacement of serotonin from tissues by a specific antimetabolite.* Science 127, 281—282 (1958).

Yagi, K., T. Nagatsu, and T. Ozawa: *Inhibitory action of chlorpromazine on the oxidation of D-amino-acid in the diencephalon part of the brain.* Nature 177, 891—892 (1956).

—, T. Ozawa, M. Ando, and T. Nagatsu: *The effect of flavin dinucleotide on the electroencephalogram modified by chlorpromazine.* J. Neurochem. 5, 304—306 (1960).

Zbinden, G., A. Pletscher u. A. Studer: *Regionäre Unterschiede der Reserpinwirkung auf enterochromaffine Zellen und 5-Hydroxytryptamin-Gehalt im Magendarmtrakt.* Schweiz. med. Wschr. 87, 629—631 (1957 a).

— — — *Hemmung der Reserpin-bedingten 5-Hydroxytryptamin-Freisetzung im enterochromaffinen System durch Isopropyl-Isonicotinsäurehydrazid.* Klin. Wschr. 35, 565—567 (1957 b).

—, u. A. Studer: *Histochemische Untersuchungen über den Einfluß von Iproniazid (Marsilid) auf die durch Reserpin erzeugte Freisetzung von Adrenalin und Noradrenalin aus dem Nebennierenmark.* Experientia 14, 201—203 (1958).

—, and L. O. Randall: *Pharmacology of Benzodiazepines: Laboratory and Clinical Correlation.* In: Advances in Pharmacology, Vol. V. Eds. S. Garattini and P. A. Shore. New York: Academic Press 1967.

—, R. E. Bagdon, E. F. Keith, R. D. Phillips, and L. O. Randall: *Experimental and clinical toxicology of chlordiazepoxide (Librium®).*

Zeller, E. A., and J. Barsky: *In vivo inhibition of liver and brain monoamine oxidase by 1-isonicotinyl-2-isopropyl-hydrazine.* Proc. Soc. exp. Biol. Med. 81, 459—461 (1952).

— —, and E. R. Berman: *Amine oxidases. XI. Inhibition of monoamine oxidase by 1-isonicotinyl-2-isopropylhydrazine.* J. Biol. Chem. 214, 267—274 (1955).

—, and J. R. Fouts: *Enzymes as primary targets of drugs.* Ann. Rev. Pharmacol. 3, 9—32 (1963).

Zetler, G., u. E. Moog: *Die Bulbocapnin-Katatonie, ihre Synergisten und Antagonisten.* Naunyn-Schmiedeberg Arch. exp. Path. 232, 442—458 (1958).

— *Pharmakologische Eigenschaften antidepressiv wirkender Pharmaka.* Dtsch. med. Wschr. 85, 2276—2281 (1960).

—, K. Mahler u. F. Daniel: *Versuche zu einer pharmakologischen Differenzierung kataleptischer Wirkungen.* Naunyn-Schmiedeberg Arch. exp. Path. 238, 486 bis 501 (1960).

Zettler, F.: *Erfahrungen mit der potenzierten Narkose und dem künstlichen Winterschlaf.* Münch. med. Wschr. 95, 1295—1296 (1953).

Zipf, H. F., u. R. Alstädter: *Die hypnotische Wirkung von Luminal und Evipan in Kombinationen mit Megaphen und anderen Phenothiazin-Derivaten.* Arzneimittelforschung 4, 14—19 (1954).

Zirkle, C. L., and C. Kaiser: *Monoamine oxidase inhibitors (nonhydrazines).* In: Psychopharmacological agents, Vol. I. Ed. M. Gordon. New York-London: Academic Press 1964, pp. 445—554.

Zirkle, G. A., P. D. King, O. B. McAtee, and R. Van Dyke: *Effects of chlorpromazine and alcohol on coordination and judgment.* J. Amer. med. Ass. 171, 1496—1499 (1959).

Type-setting, printing and binding:
Konrad Triltsch, Graphischer Betrieb, 87 Würzburg, Germany